"Callanetics is a way of life that enriches and strengthens your body, mind, and spirit. It is what I call a *cross-training tool* to enhance the skills you already possess. If you already jog or swim or dance, Callanetics will help you jog or swim or dance better; if you sing, Callanetics will improve your voice and your lung power; if you are tense and tired, Callanetics will revitalize your energy.

"I hope this book will help you reclaim your life and your vitality, and find yourself on the road to being fit forever."

—Callan Pinckney

• • • • • • • • • •

CALLAN PINCKNEY, *fifty-six, is the author of the* New York Times *bestseller* Callanetics, *and of* Super Callanetics, Callanetics Countdown, *and* Callanetics for Your Back. *Her bestselling videos include* Callanetics *(a* Billboard *bestseller for six years),* Beginning Callanetics, Super Callanetics, AM/PM Callanetics, *and the* Quick Callanetics *series. Callanetics is taught by certified instructors in franchised studios around the world. Callan lives in Savannah, Georgia.*

OTHER BOOKS BY CALLAN PINCKNEY

Callanetics

Callanetics for Your Back

Callanetics Countdown

Super Callanetics

CALLANETICS FIT FOREVER

By Callan Pinckney

A PERIGEE BOOK

A Perigee Book
Published by The Berkley Publishing Group
A division of Penguin Putnam Inc.
375 Hudson Street
New York, New York 10014

Copyright © 1995 by Callan Pinckney
Book design by Mauna Eichner
Cover Design by Isabella Fasciano
Front and back cover photographs © 1995 by Anthony Loew

First G. P. Putnam's Sons edition: January 1996
First Perigee edition: January 1997
Perigee ISBN: 0-399-52263-8

Published simultaneously in Canada.

The Penguin Putnam Inc. World Wide Web site address is
http://www.penguinputnam.com

The Library of Congress has catalogued the G. P. Putnam's Sons edition as follows:

Pinckney, Callan.
    Callanetics fit forever / by Callan Pinckney.
        p.   cm.
    ISBN 0-399-14121-9
    Includes index.
    1. Exercise for women.   2. Middle-aged women – Health and hygiene.
        3. Physical fitness for women.   I. Title.
    RA781.P5753   1996   95-31928   CIP
    613.7'045 – dc20

Printed in the United States of America

10   9   8   7   6   5   4   3

CONTENTS

PART I · FIT FOREVER

. . . .

2. Strengthen Your Heart   29

. . . .

3. Eating Healthy   45

4. Stress and How to Get Rid of It   93

PART II   CALLANETICS EXERCISES

5. Callanetics   127

6. CardioCallanetics

7. Special Routines and Maintenance Plans

ACKNOWLEDGMENTS

I am especially grateful to Pat Klein, president of the Callanetics Management Company, Laurie Shanahan, and Kathleen Horstmeyer; as well as the marvelous Ruth Jeffries and Lynne Marotta of the Callanetics Studio of Manhattan; exercise pro Sara Kooperman; and photographer Paul Sherman.

This book could not have been completed without the expert editorial guidance of Karen Moline. Special thanks are also due to Ellen M. Laura, a certified Callanetics teacher, for her generous permission to use excerpts from her forthcoming book, *The Most Fattening Thing You Can Do Is Go on a Diet*. Her nutritional expertise helped shape much of chapter 3, particularly the Eat with a Plan and Shop with a Plan sections and many dietary tips. I would also like to thank Cheryl Hartsough, R.D., L.D., dietitian and nutritionist at the PGA Spa, for her useful tips on how and what to eat; Shirley Babior, L.C.S.W., at The Center for Anxiety and Stress Treatment in San Diego, California, and Tina Van De Graaf, L.M.T., assistant spa director at the PGA Spa in Palm Beach, Florida, for their invaluable tips about combating stress; and Dr. Margaret Moline, director of the Sleep-Wake Disorders Center of the New York Hospital-Cornell Medical Center, for her expert information about insomnia. Special thanks to the indefatigable agents Mitch Douglas and Suzanne Gluck at ICM, and to my attorney, Marc L. Bailin, for his continued help and support.

A NOTE OF WARNING

The exercise programs contained herein are intended for persons in good health. Before beginning these or any other exercise programs, it is essential to obtain the approval and recommendations of your physician. It is suggested that you read through the text once to become familiar with the exercises before beginning these programs.

IF YOU ARE PREGNANT

If you are pregnant, *under no circumstances* should you do the Open and Close exercises. If you are a woman in the first trimester of pregnancy, under no circumstances should you attempt the stomach exercises in this book. After the first trimester it may be safe for you to do these exercises gently, but clear this with your doctor first. Do not do any of these exercises unless your doctor has actually tried and experienced them personally before giving approval. Showing your doctor this book is not enough. Insist that he or she do the exercises to feel how deep the contractions are. At first glance, these exercises appear to be very easy, but in fact they may be too powerful to be performed during pregnancy.

A NOTE ABOUT DIET AND NUTRITION

The nutrition and diet material in this book is based upon current research that is often contradictory in nature. Although the nutrition and diet material contained in this book is based upon information from the most commonly held theories available at the time of this writing, users should not embark upon these or any other diet or nutritional programs without first consulting a physician as to how they might apply to them.

CALLANETICS FIT FOREVER

From "Fit Forever": (30 Days To A Beautiful Body)

warm ups

Underarm Tightener	100		p. 134
Waist Away	100		p. 135
Neck Stretch	5	R to L in triple slow ____	
Neck Roll	5		p. 137

Stomach

Bent Knee Reach	100		p. 138
Single Leg Raise	100		p. 139
Double Leg Raise	100		p. 141
Both Legs Over	60	hands above head "乙 o 丁" legs over to side	
Neck To Side	1	ear to shoulder hold 15 both sides	
3/4 Neck Relaxer	1	chin to 1/2 between neck + shoulder hold 15 curl pelvis	

Legs And Inner Thighs

Bend And Curl	10 (1" at a time)	p. 142 (only 5)	
Plié And Balance	20 (lower 6")	p. 143 (only 10)	
Up And Over	60	p. 143 (only 50)	
Hamstring Stretch	100	p. 149 (only 50)	
Standing Stretch	60	stand at bar, curl pelvis, hold foot behind you	
Inner Thigh Tightener	100	p. 155	

Buttocks, Hips, And Outer Thighs

Bringing Up The Rear	100	p. 144	
Out To The Side	100	p. 145	
Pelvic Circles	5	p. 151	
Pelvic Dip	5	p. 152	
Front Thigh Stretch	40	p. 154	
Crossover	60	p. 150	

INTRODUCTION

You're Not Getting Older, You're Getting Better

America is obsessed with aging. Or should I say, America is obsessed with *not* aging. Women are not supposed to get old. Skinny teenage models sell us wrinkle cream. Even skinnier teenage models show us clothes and bodies we can never hope to have. Sixty-year-old male movie stars have movie wives half their age. Cosmetic surgery is booming. Yet . . .

No one I've ever met says she wants to get older, yet America is also a country that is, like it or not, getting older. In thirty-five years more than 20 percent of Americans will be over the age of sixty-five. And at the rate we're going, most of them will be passive, unhappy, unhealthy blobs. One out of every two Americans will die from heart disease. Cancer strikes three out of four families. Almost twelve million Americans have diabetes, and fifty-eight million have hypertension. At least 40 percent of all Americans are overweight, and 25 percent are obese; for women this means their bodies are more than 30 percent fat. This means their children are learning bad eating habits, getting fatter and tired and suffering from low self-esteem about their appearance, setting themselves up for a lifetime of health problems. And with the health-care crisis looming large, we all need to face facts about our health and who's going to pay for taking care of it.

Our bodies are designed to be active, throughout our entire lives. But we've reduced our physical activity by nearly 75 percent since 1900. We know more about dieting and exercise and reasons to keep fit than ever—and yet we keep getting fatter and fatter. Obesity doesn't only mean that you look fat. Obesity is actually a disease that greatly increases your probability of developing heart disease, cancer, diabetes, and many other ailments, as well as an endless cycle of self-criticism and doubt.

When was the last time you felt strong, vital, and healthy?

This is where Callanetics can help you. It's so easy to forget that the most incredible exercise machine ever invented is your own wonderful body. I found that out when I invented Callanetics, and now at the age of fifty-seven, I am stronger, more vital, and healthier than I've ever been.

Callanetics is a way of life that enriches and strengthens your body, mind, and spirit. It is what I call a *cross-training tool* to enhance the skills you already possess. If you already jog or swim or dance, Callanetics will help you jog or swim or dance better; if you sing, Callanetics will improve your voice and your lung power; if you are tense and tired, Callanetics will revitalize your energy. So many of my students were resistant to any discussion about weight because they'd been told so many times (and by so many people) that the reason they were fat is because they're lazy. These people discovered that Callanetics worked where other programs had failed because it taught them to proceed at their own pace, and was entirely nonjudgmental. Every tiny bit of progress was cause for celebration.

How Callanetics Works

Callanetics is a revolutionary, nonimpact exercise program that tones and reshapes your body. The exercises consist of small, delicate movements with no jarring or straining to stress your joints. You can feel the difference in minutes and see the dramatic results after a few short sessions.

I developed Callanetics because it was a matter of sheer survival. I was born with scoliosis (curvature of the spine), bad feet, and other medical problems. Despite that, I was able to study and excel at the ballet I loved. In my twenties, I spent years hitchhiking and traveling around the world, carrying all my belongings in a sixty-two-pound rucksack. As a result, doctors told me to have immediate surgery on my knees and back because they were such a mess! Motivated by pain, I spent ages experimenting with exercise techniques to ease my aches, and this gradually turned into Callanetics, and I turned into a teacher. In 1984 I published *Callanetics*, which spent a year on the *New York Times* best-seller list.

I've since published *Callanetics for Your Back, Super Callanetics, Callanetics Countdown* books and audiotapes, as well as *Callanetics, Super Callanetics, AM/PM Callanetics, 3 Quick Callanetics,* and *Beginning Callanetics* exercise videos to help you practice at home. There are dozens of Callanetics studios around America, offering classes to thousands of people looking for help—and finding it!

As a teacher one of the most gratifying aspects is observing students improve so quickly, to see their amazement when they become stronger and more toned—to watch their attitude go from "I Can't" to "Look at Me." One of my students was a woman in her sixties who was so unused to any sort of physical activity that she could hardly move a muscle. In fact, when she first came to class she could barely raise her hands over her head—much less think about holding on to the barre or hanging. Well, by her seventh class she was hanging, enjoying that lovely stretch, and pleased as punch about it. I literally watched her blossom. She so quickly learned how to undo the bad habits of a lifetime, to *work at her own pace,* and *listen to her body.* Most of all, she learned how to *relax.*

Callanetics Can Work When Other Exercise Regimes Fail

One of the aspects of Callanetics that is the most difficult to explain to someone who hasn't tried these fabulous exercises is the unique importance of the way we stretch. Most people think that you must tense your muscles to strengthen them. Callanetics teaches you how to *relax* to *strengthen* these muscles.

If you take Callanetics classes you already know that we strive to create a very calm, nurturing environment. The first thing you learn is how wrong the No Pain, No Gain concept really is. You don't have to suffer to get stronger. We don't allow negativism in our students, and we certainly don't allow any kind of competition. There are no exercise addicts showing off their designer workout gear and state-of-the-art shoes—there are no shoes, period! So many women come to Callanetics after being frustrated (by the frenetic pace) or embarrassed (by the smug attitude of the perky little gym bunnies half their age) or injured (by high-impact classes) at their local gym or fitness center. They first arrive wearing baggy sweats and voluminous T-shirts because they can't stand to look at their bodies . . . but as soon as they see results—which are usually immediate—the next thing you know, there's a new leotard and a whole new attitude.

We're so used to criticizing our bodies and putting ourselves down, but Callanetics teaches you to have no self-consciousness and no self-doubt about what you can do. It teaches you to *listen to your body* and *always work at your own pace.* You'll quickly gain respect for your body. As your body strengthens, you learn how to move. And how to *feel.* This can be a tremendously empowering experience for so many of us who've spent a lifetime unable to let go of our fears and worries about our capabilities.

How Callanetics Is Unique

- These exercises are not like standard exercises—because they involve deep muscular contracting and stretching at the same time. The more you contract, the more you work your muscles. Callanetics stretches elongate your muscless.

- Callanetics improves your flexibility. Sports physiologists agree that stretching is one of the most neglected yet essential components of any exercise regime. Yogis say that you're only as young as your spine . . . and that the more flexibility in your spine, the more there is in your mind. I couldn't agree more!

- These exercises are not like many other strengthening programs—because they create long, lean muscles, not large, bulky, beefy ones. The more lean muscle you have, the more you increase your metabolic rate, which means you'll burn more calories, whether exercising, working, or resting.

- These exercises are not like ballet or yoga—because they do not take years to perfect and involve no difficult or unusual positions.

- You don't need any special equipment or clothing or shoes—only a chair or sofa. You can do them any time of the day, at home or even in your office.

- These exercises are not like any other—because they give you results so quickly, without fear of injury. They involve no strenuous breathing and sweating. You can do them at lunchtime and then go back to work refreshed.

- Callanetics helps you defy gravity. Your jawline will tighten and your double chins will disappear; your breasts will be lifted up; you will actually sculpt your thighs and bottom. As one of my students said, Callanetics is like a face-lift for your body.

- Callanetics uniquely teaches you how to isolate your large muscle groups and use your body properly. It is capable of so much more than you ever imagined! This wonderful sense of body awareness will stay with you for the rest of your life.

- Most of all, the unique movements of Callanetics strengthen and relax you at the same time. No longer will you feel exhausted or drained after a workout. You'll feel energized and empowered.

My Fitness Philosophy

These are words you'll hear over and over again when you do Callanetics:

- Always work at your own pace.
- Listen to your body.
- Never, ever force.
- Relax your entire body.
- Light and flowing as a feather.
- Triple slow motion.
- Never compare yourself with anyone else.

These words will become part of your life, no matter what you're doing. They're equally important for exercise, meals, work and play, family life, or time spent alone.

My fitness philosophy is to work with what you have. There's always room for improvement. No one—certainly not me—has a perfect body. No one has a perfect life. We have to find the right balance to make ourselves healthy, happy, and productive.

Consistency is the key. That's why fad diets don't work and never have. That's why we're all confused. We simply don't know what to believe with all this contradictory information. This month it's cholesterol.

Or fat grams. Eat lots of pasta and complex carbohydrates. No, don't do that—someone just discovered that pasta makes you fat. Cholesterol is bad. Whoops, forgot to tell you some forms of cholesterol are *good*. Or are they? This chart says you should weigh this much. That chart says you shouldn't. All the relaxing Callanetics exercises in the world won't make you stop screaming in frustration!

Despite the hundreds of books in your library and local bookstores, the way to stay fit forever is based on plain old common sense—putting it into motion is what's difficult. This book will show you how to combine Callanetics (which gives you strength and flexibility) with some form of aerobic exercise (which is either walking or swimming or CardioCallanetics) with a simple, low-fat diet plan.

Let me put it another way:

How to Get Old in a Hurry	How to Stay Young in a Hurry
Eat badly	Eat well
Don't exercise regularly	Exercise regularly
Smoke	Stop smoking
Sleep poorly	Sleep deeply
Drink alcohol	Drink Water
Complain about your health	Do something about your health
Feel sorry for yourself	Feel blessed to be alive

Of course I can't promise you that Callanetics or any exercise/fitness program will add years to your life, but I can promise you that exercise should improve the *quality* of your life. You can strengthen your heart and all the other muscles as well as the bones in your body no matter what your age.

How Easy It Is to Make Changes

I'm just too tired. I hear that all the time (and have often said it myself). But there are two different types of fatigue: *weariness*, when your vitality and creativity, your inner energy, seems to have drained all away; and *fa-*

tigue, when you are physically exhausted from lack of sleep, illness, poor eating, stress, overwork, etc., etc., etc.

With our hectic lives, it's so much easier to blame our problems on *fatigue*, when what's really bothering us is *weariness*. If we keep trying to resolve the problems in our lives—work, love, family, health, the leaky faucet in the kitchen—and never seem to get anywhere, we get *weary* with the frustration of it all. Taking care of everyone else and leaving no time for ourselves provoke even more frustration.

That's where Callanetics comes in. Take five, ten, fifteen minutes for yourself to practice Callanetics, and you've taken the first step to bring some relief from fatigue and weariness into your life. As you gain strength in your muscles and watch your body gradually and painlessly transform itself, confidence that has long been eroded begins to return, and frustrations seem to melt away. Exercise does that. It gets rid of tension without any negative side effects whatsoever. All the results are beneficial. The happiest people I know have a sense of purpose in life and in their goals. If you're feeling alone and unhappy, it's so easy to give in and say, well, What does one more day of bad eating and bad habits have to do with anything?

If you stick with Callanetics, your body *will* change shape, your energy *will* increase, and your motivation to stick to a regime *will not* leave you as so many other programs have before.

If you've been like so many of us and have used the wrong strategy to get thin—deprivation dieting without exercise—you're probably frustrated (and hungry). Callanetics exercise will cut your appetite and help you shed your deprivation mentality and gradually shift priorities until you look forward to exercising. Just one hour of Callanetics can be so rejuvenating because you feel the results every time you exercise. The exhaustion and discouragement of deprivation dieting will be replaced by an amazing sense of accomplishment. The more you do Callanetics, the more you learn how to listen to your body, how to be aware of what a wonderful creation it is.

Equally important, when you perform Callanetics you will learn how to know when to stop. You can learn to do the same thing when you eat, and when you find yourself unable to escape from all the stresses bombarding you in daily life.

Best of all, there's never an excuse *not* to do Callanetics. If it's snowing you don't have to worry about going out in the cold. If there's a heat wave, you don't have to worry about getting overheated. If you only have fifteen minutes to spare, you can do an abbreviated yet deep-working routine. If you've had knee or back problems, you won't have to worry about injuries. You see results so quickly that you won't get discouraged. Callanetics works for everyone.

How I've Modified Callanetics for Older Women

As I'll detail in the next chapter, our bodies inevitably change as we age—yet they needn't inevitably change for the worst. Chances are, of course, that as our lives progress we suffer more injuries and illnesses; tend to have metabolisms that slow down, weight that piles on, and bones that break because we don't exercise. Often our circumstances change—especially as we become less active (if you're retired, for example, you naturally won't be expending the same amount of energy if you're spending more time in the house than at work). Somehow we begin to think that, inevitably, we *must* have to live with aches and pains and discomfort.

Older women are often stuck in a situation where their lack of fitness and years of living in overweight bodies not only embarrass them but make them want to give up, convinced that they'll never be able to find a workout regime that is safe and effective for their needs, and that the state of their bodies makes it either too difficult or too painful to even want to try. But once your doctor has given you the go-ahead to start exercising, Callanetics are ideal for those who've been unable to follow any other program. Because it is gentle, respectful to older bodies, and perfectly safe for even those who have never exercised before to do Callanetics every day, these exercises are especially practical for those who are new to working out, or live in rural areas where there are no gyms or fitness centers. With either my books or videos as your guide, you do these exercises in your own time and at your own pace. Callanetics will help you become in touch with your body. You will learn how to *feel*, how to release all the tension that's been stored in your body not only from a hard day's work but from years of not knowing how to release it.

In the second part of this book, you'll find the perfect Callanetics routine to do no matter what your age, shape, size, or medical condition.

You'll be increasing your muscle strength with each hour that you perform these exercises and will find it amazingly simple to maintain your new figure with ease because you only need a few sessions per week to stay tight and toned.

CardioCallanetics

For optimal health, our bodies need aerobic exercise. "Aerobic" means "with oxygen." (Callanetics exercises themselves are "anaerobic," which means "without oxygen.") Any form of aerobic exercise done over a minimum of twenty minutes—a brisk walk or jog, bike ride or swim, dancing or stair stepping—will strengthen your cardiovascular system, your muscles, and help you burn fat.

CardioCallanetics increases your heart rate like all aerobic exercise, but it feels different. That's because it's the logical next step for Callanetics—using the concept of meditation in motion—and putting you into motion! CardioCallanetics helps you develop stamina, maintain the well-being of your heart and decrease the risk of heart disease, burn fat, and invigorate your mind and body.

As you'll see in chapter 6, CardioCallanetics is low-impact aerobic exercise that is easy to follow. (High-impact exercises can burn calories and fat but can seriously damage your knees, back, and neck.) It will challenge you without any discomfort or stress. You'll be letting the natural rhythms of your body move you—and you'll have so much fun with it, you won't want to stop!

You'll also be burning up fat by increasing your physical-activity level. Think of it this way: to lose weight sensibly, you'll want to be able to eat enough to feel full—not deprived—so you'll be able to reach your goal. If you're eating an average of 2,500 calories a day and you reduce this to 2,000, you can be quite sure that you'll lose one pound per week. But if you reduce your calories by only 250 (which is one cup of ice cream) and increase your physical activity by 250 calories (which is one-half hour of brisk walking or jogging), you'll also lose one pound per week, build muscle, feel stronger, decrease your appetite, and have more energy. What sounds better?

If you need any more convincing, look at Oprah Winfrey. She slimmed down to a remarkable size ten on a liquid diet—and it all came back and then some, with a vengeance. Oprah finally realized that her obesity would not go away on a starvation diet; nor would her weight *stay* off unless she combined a low-fat diet with a consistent exercise program. She hired her own cook and found the discipline within herself to stick with a workout program. And she looks better than ever—slim, fit, and strong.

But how many of us can afford our own chefs to prepare tasty low-cal meals for us every day of the week? (I'd settle for one breakfast in bed!) How many can afford a personal trainer to force us to jog one more mile? Not many. But don't let that discourage you.

There's an old Chinese proverb: "Can do—do. Can't do—still learning." If you wake up every day and say to yourself, "I know what I need to do, and I just have to do it . . . but I'll think about it tomorrow," that attitude is like a locked door barricading the path between you and your goals. Your thoughts cannot change unless you have new ideas, unless you are receptive to learning and growing all your life.

Becoming healthy and rethinking long-established patterns of eating and behaving is a new skill. It is a learnable skill, but it's not—like any skill worth learning—an immediate or overnight sensation. There is no magic potion involved to instantly make you slim and fit (or young and rich!), only a little bit of learning and practice.

Callanetics will teach you how to become unconsciously competent. It's like learning how to drive a stick-shift car. The first time you drive, it's practically impossible to get out of first gear; after a few driving sessions, you don't even have to think about it. Eating and exercise are no different. After you practice and change not only what you're eating but how you think about it, you'll realize that you aren't weighing and measuring food servings anymore. You aren't eating everything on your plate simply because it's there. You aren't craving pints of ice cream and raiding the fridge in the middle of the night. You aren't thinking compulsively about food. You aren't making excuses not to go work out. You're simply doing it.

So many of my students have watched me in class and asked me, "Callan, how do you *do* that?" The only thing I can say is that I just get in the position and relax. My body knows what to do. Callanetics is my heart and soul, and because I've been doing it for so long I have become unconsciously competent at it. Believe me, if I can become competent at Callanetics, at maintaining my fitness after a lifetime of back and foot problems, you can also. I'm not a model or an actress. I'm a teacher. It's certainly my job as a teacher to give you lessons on how not to turn into a little old lady who lets herself be defeated by life and her body. I've had seventy-two-year-old women come into class and say to me, *"Please, tell me it's too late. Tell me I can go home. Tell me I'm weak."* Of course I tell them nothing of the sort!

One of the very hardest things I've ever learned how to do is give up my rigidity, manifested by my chronic back and foot problems, because I was in so much pain and too scared to open up and expose my vulnerable self to a new world of *feeling*. Despite my travels around the world and all the wonderful, crazy experiences I'd had, I still had to teach myself how to take risks, how to say this is what I want, this is what's good for me. To be able to say I don't know and ask for help. To be able to *listen to my body*.

Age doesn't matter. Some of the most youthful, vital people I've met are "old" in age only. They see life as an adventure. They know that you're only as old as you feel, and it's never too late to awaken to all the possibilities life has to offer. If you give up and let yourself feel old, you'll start to believe it, and then you will be old—it's a self-fulfilling prophecy.

Callanetics is a never-ending process of learning—like addictive meditation. I hope this book will begin to help you reclaim your life and your vitality, and find yourself on the road to being fit forever.

FIT FOREVER

HOW YOUR BODY CHANGES AS YOU AGE

It's Never Too Late: Why More Than Ever We Need to Keep Fit

Every living creature is part of the cycle of birth, growth, maturity, and aging. But in our youth-oriented society, the very thought of aging scares us because we equate it with inevitable decline and then death. Pessimists can look at aging this way:

1. Our bones become more fragile. This means our bones break. By the age of ninety, as many as 32 percent of women will have broken their hips (and 12 to 20 percent will die from complications suffered after a broken hip).

2. Our muscles become less strong. For each decade after the age of twenty-five, we lose 3 to 5 percent of our muscle mass. This means we become progressively weaker.

3. Our joints become less mobile. This means we become much less flexible.

4. Our bone and muscle body weight declines but our body fat increases.

5. Our immune system, which protects us from disease and infection, works less efficiently, which means we become sicker.

6. Our skin loses elasticity, changing from smooth to wrinkled, and our hair thins and turns gray.

7. Our memory begins to lapse, and our vision and hearing decline.

8. We get very discouraged. We lose sexual desire. We feel old, so we act old.

Yet optimists look at aging another way: gaining a lifetime of experience and wisdom. Every single item on this list can be combated with Callanetics Fit Forever.

Changes in Metabolism

What exactly is metabolism?

The dictionary says that metabolism is the total of all the chemical processes that convert food into the energy for the maintenance of your body. This is a constant process. Whether you are sleeping, reading, vacuuming, working, making love, or eating, you're burning calories. (When you're sitting in front of the television, you're burning the least amount of calories possible in a waking state.) Food converted to energy is expressed in calories, and the total number of calories used each day is our metabolic rate. In other words our *metabolic rate* is basically how quickly our body burns calories.

Our metabolism peaks at age twenty-four, then decreases with age because our muscles decrease with age. If your muscles are basically unused, they need less oxygen, and you need fewer calories. According to Dr. William Evans, coauthor of the book *Biomarkers: The 10 Determinants of Aging You Can Control*, "Based on our estimates of the average loss of lean-body mass with age, a person's basal metabolism drops about 2 percent per decade starting at age twenty." Therefore, if you're the average American couch potato, you'll have a low metabolic rate, and your body will be primed to store all your excess calories as fat.

When you are thin and fit, your body is lean and muscled. Don't believe what our gym teachers might have erroneously told us all those years ago about muscles being bad for our figures: Muscles, on women, are good. Muscle is metabolically active tissue, even when we're not doing anything active. Muscles burn more than two-thirds of all the energy we use. Muscle weighs more, so that your scale may tell you that you haven't "lost weight," yet your dress size has gone down a notch or two. The more the muscle, the higher the metabolism. A strong body can take in more food because muscles constantly need calories just to maintain themselves. Fat doesn't. It just sits there, inert, making your life (and health) a misery.

Must You Gain Weight?

Of course not. But if you sit on your behind all day at work, then you come home and collapse in front of the TV with a bag of potato chips and a pint of ice cream, yes, of course you're going to gain weight.

How to slow down your metabolism:

> Don't exercise.
>
> Go on starvation, deprivation, very low-calorie diets.

I guarantee that if you do both of the above, you'll not only gain weight when you start eating normally again, but you'll feel tired, sluggish, and just plain blah.

> If you don't exercise, your metabolism slows down and your body burns fewer calories.
>
> When you gain weight back, it is stored as fat.

Dr. Rudolph Leibel, a researcher at Rockefeller University, recently discovered that every body has what he calls a "set point," or natural weight. You can't change this tendency any more than you can change your height or body type, which helps explain why some people are naturally thin and others, who really don't eat a lot, tend to be heavier. If your weight goes below this set point, mostly due to a deprivation kind of diet, your metabolism slows and you burn less fat. When your weight goes above it, your metabolism speeds up and burns more fat.

Knowing that your body has a set point of natural weight that might be higher than you'd like it is no excuse to overeat and not exercise. You *can* make your metabolism more efficient, no matter what your age. The key is to burn lots of calories all day, not just when you're exercising. The important factor is to build enough muscle to raise your metabolic rate higher than ever.

For example, let's use 1,000 calories. By raising your metabolic rate by 1,000 calories—from, let's say, 1,500 to 2,500 calories a day—you would burn 1,000 more calories per day. It takes about five hours of exercise to burn 1,000 calories. It's a lot easier to build muscle that will burn this 1,000 calories for you than to exercise five hours a day.

And how do you do that?

1. Do your Callanetics exercises, because they increase your muscle strength without building bulk. Strength training adds calorie-burning and body-toning muscle as it helps you lose fat. And when your muscle tone is improved, your body is toned and fit. This can do wonders for not only your appearance but also your self-esteem. (See part 2.)

2. Incorporate some form of aerobic exercise into your life. If you exercise regularly, you can lose weight by eating *more* calories than if you were just dieting. Not only that, exercise makes you feel good not only when you're doing it (and burning calories) but also for hours afterwards. Don't let anyone who doesn't exercise tell you it can't be fun! (See chapter 2.)

3. Learn to rethink your eating patterns. You don't have to be overweight and miserable about it. (See chapter 3.)

4. Unload the stress that's weighing you down. Callanetics exercises are what I call meditation in motion. (See chapter 4.)

The Difference Between Muscles and Fat

There are three basic body types, and no matter how much exercise we do or how well we eat, we can't ever change the shape of our bones.

Human beings are either endomorphs (round and curvaceous like Marilyn Monroe), mesomorphs (larger bones and natural athletes like Madonna), or ectomorphs (lean and slender build like models). Endomorphs tend toward high body fat and often have a hard time losing weight; mesomorphs can also become quite thick around the middle; and ectomorphs may look thin even though they may have a high body fat to muscle ratio. (Believe me, if you see enough fashion shows, you'll realize that the super-skinny models are often surprisingly flabby. They're going to be in for an unpleasant surprise as they get older and start piling on the pounds!)

If you are an endomorph or mesomorph, you'll tend to put weight on as either an "apple" (around your midsection), or a "pear" (around your hips and buttocks). Unfortunately, "apples" are predisposed to have a higher risk for heart disease, hypertension, and diabetes than "pears" are, so they've really got to be extra careful about their weight.

Regretfully, our society has decided that thin, bony, and boyish is the way we're supposed to look, even though the vast majority of women can't possibly hope to achieve this silhouette. The increasing number of young girls who are on "diets" are setting themselves up for a lifetime of eating disorders and misery.

But what, exactly, is your body made of? Your body weight is a combination of water, muscle, bones, organs, tissues, and, of course, FAT. Every body has a different proportion of these components, so if you have large bones, you'll naturally have more "bone weight" than someone who is petite. Body composition is more accurate than body weight for determining how healthy you are.

As those of us who used to be compulsive scale-watchers know, the scale weight can fluctuate on a daily basis—but the scale can't tell you if you've lost or gained water, or fat, or muscle. Especially as muscle weighs twice as much as fat!

How often have we said, Oh well, I *used* to exercise, but when I stopped the muscle turned to fat. The truth is that fat cells and muscle cells are completely different and can't be changed from one into the other. Fat cells store and release fat, and muscle cells create energy to move our bodies. During aerobic exercise, muscle cells metabolize energy and use stored fat—provided by the fat cells. Since these two functions happen simultaneously, we mistakenly think that fat is being transformed into muscle. What really happens is that muscle cells are *re-*

placing the fat cells. Of course if we stop exercising, the opposite occurs. Muscle cells burn less energy so fat cells store more fat than they release.

According to fitness expert Ellen Laura, to find out what shape your body really is in, you'll need to know roughly your body fat percentage. Here are the ranges:

14–17 percent	Very low fat, ultralean = athletes
17–20	Low fat, slim = models
21–24	Healthy = recommended range
25–29	Above recommended range = trouble
29–35	High fat = overfat
35 percent plus	Very high fat = obese

The most accurate measurements of body fat are done by professionals—but remember, at best these are only estimates. (The only truly accurate way to measure body fat is to melt down your body, skim off the fat, and then measure it. That sounds rather drastic, doesn't it!) A trained technician can either take skin-fold measurements with a special caliper, or weigh you underwater (body weight on land divided by the loss of body weight in the water); or use what's called Bioelectrical Impedence Analysis, where a painless electric current measures resistance. There's also a new at-home scale, made by the Tanita Corporation, but at $550, it's a bit too expensive for nearly everyone. (Call 1-800-Tanita-8 for more information.)

A simple test can be done at home with a "pinch-an-inch" test. Midway between your elbow and shoulder, pinch your skin with your forefinger and thumb. Then pinch at your stomach, then midway between your right hip bone and navel, and measure.

Upper Arm and Stomach	Score
More than 1½ inches	Poor
1–1½ inches	Fair
½ inch	Good
Less than ½ inch	Excellent

Here's a typical dieting scenario my colleague Ellen M. Laura uses to help explain what body-fat percentages really mean: Mary Smith is 5 feet 6 inches and weighs 135 pounds when she graduates from college and begins her job as a computer programmer. When she'd been a student, she played lots of sports and had hour-long aerobic and weight-training sessions at the gym at least three times a week. Her body fat was a healthy 20 percent.

Let's visit Mary ten years later. She's gained 10 pounds, so she weighs 145. Right?

Wrong. The scale says 145, but the scale can't differentiate among muscle, fat, and water weight. In reality, Mary has *lost* 5 pounds of muscle because she stopped exercising. That means she's *gained* 15 pounds of fat! Her body fat is now 29 percent of her total body weight.

And so Mary does what most of us would do: she goes on a strict diet. (But she leaves out the crucial fat-burning edge—and neglects to exercise.) After two months of suffering and starvation, Mary is thrilled to have lost those 10 pesky pounds. She'd be much less thrilled to learn that she's lost 7 pounds of fat and 3 pounds of muscle, bringing her body fat to 26 percent, which is still in the unhealthy range. Worst of all, her metabolism has slowed because she has less active tissue—muscle—so when she starts eating normally again, she'll gradually gain back all her weight as *fat*. Her body fat percentage is now a whopping 31, and she's flabbier and more miserable than ever.

Not only that, but Mary doesn't know that her fat cells have two sets of enzymes, which are substances in your body that cause reactions to take place. There are fat-storing, or lipogenic, enzymes and fat-releasing, or lipolytic, enzymes. Each time we start a diet, our body is tricked into thinking there's a famine, so it strives to make its metabolism more efficient and actually burns fewer calories. It also creates more fat-storing enzymes so that when the famine—your diet—is over, it will be able to store fat even more efficiently in case there's another famine.

So, if a normal fit woman eats dessert, her fat-releasing enzymes get to work digesting her food. But when a fat woman eats dessert, her fat-*storing* enzymes get to work. It's a double whammy. Fat people not only have less lean in their bodies, but they also have more fat-*storing* enzymes to burn the fat they *do* eat less efficiently.

The way to change all that is to rethink the way we eat, breathe, and move.

That Aching Back/Those Creaking Joints . . . Needn't Be a Pain

Do you know what the number-one disability for people under forty-five is? Low back pain and back injuries, mostly caused by muscle and tendon sprains that send our muscles into spasms and us screaming into the night. According to the American Academy of Orthopedic Surgeons, at least 80 million Americans have had or are now suffering from back pain. Medical experts also say that low back pain is the most expensive benign health condition in this country, and the reason why is the simple (and awful) fact that we are pathetically out of shape and overweight. Most back pain is not caused by disease but by a problem with our vertebrae, discs, ligaments, and muscles, usually due to poor posture at work and in our cars, strain on our backs (our own body weight), and bending. That's why I wrote *Callanetics for Your Back,* and I strongly urge you to use that book if you have any back pain, because it can help since it's full of exercises and advice to help alleviate your suffering. Of course you should always see a doctor or chiropractor for diagnoses and treatment as well. I also recommend acupuncture for pain relief, hot packs and baths, and massage (if your problem is caused by muscle spasms and not your vertebrae or discs).

Your spine is made up of twenty-four flexible yet stable vertebrae, the sacrum, and the tailbone, or coccyx. This column protects your spinal cord from injury. In between each vertebra is a *disc,* made of tough fibers and cartilage with a jellylike center. As we age, our discs become smaller, less resilient and effective, and cause problems. This makes us very vulnerable to any strenuous, sudden, or twisting movements. Sciatica is also a common problem, a swelling or injury to the sciatic nerve, which causes pain, soreness, or tingling. The sciatic nerve starts at the base of the spine and travels down the back of the thigh and leg to the foot, which means that the pain can be relentless.

Lower back pain tends to come along the older we get but that's usually through an accumulation of all our bad habits. We can throw our back out lifting, bending, and vacuuming. We can ache from sitting at our desks all day in uncomfortable chairs. We don't realize how the vibrations in our car can injure us. We can wince from too much coughing from too much smoking. We can twinge from stress and anxiety and poor posture. We can throb from too much tennis or golf or any other sport that makes us twist and turn. But this doesn't mean you have to suffer from back pain all your life.

Since more than 80 percent of lower back pain is caused by weak or tense muscles, you can start taking immediate steps to get stronger. If you're physically fit, exercise regularly—especially those pesky abdominal muscles—and take care of yourself, chances are you can banish most back pain from your life. Easier said than done!

Here are a few hints to avoid back pain:

Sit straight. Be aware of your posture, no matter where you are.

When lifting and carrying, hold items close to your body. Always bend from your knees.

Lose weight. It's straining your back.

Let go of stress, especially if you automatically "stiffen" your spine when upset.

Deep breathing exercises can help.

Support your back while driving and when at work. Many of us are forced to work in offices that are not designed correctly (the science of designing objects that work for us is called ergonomics), so that we're not sitting in chairs that properly brace us, or we're forced to sit at work stations that are misproportioned for our height. If you work at a keyboard or factory or cash register, this can cause repetitive stress disorder and/or carpal tunnel syndrome in your wrists and hands in addition to stressing your whole body. Make sure your work chair is adjustable. Prop up special cushions or pillows behind your back when you drive. Get up and stretch often.

Once you master Callanetics, your back will automatically strengthen. You'll know how to get up off the floor (see p. 131)... you'll know how to float like a feather... you'll know how to walk tall and proud... You'll remember to bend your knees whenever you pick anything up... and you'll know how important it is to have strong, firm abdominal muscles giving you a taut belly and helping to support your back. You'll also know how the Pelvic Wave can help banish back pain and release tension nearly instantly.

Diseases: Cancer, Heart Disease, Diabetes, and Alzheimer's

Cancer

Cancer is a group of diseases that have one thing in common: groups of unwanted cells multiplying out of control. Caught early enough, cancer can usually be cured by a combination of surgery, chemotherapy, and radiation therapy.

According to the American Cancer Society, these are the warning signs of cancer, spelled out by Caution:

C	Change in bowel or bladder habits
A	A sore that does not heal
U	Unusual bleeding or discharge
T	Thickening or lump in breast or any part of the body
I	Indigestion or difficulty swallowing
O	Obvious change in a wart or mole
N	Nagging cough or hoarseness.

Most cancers in their earliest, most treatable stages do not cause any symptoms or pain. That's why body awareness and self-checking as well as regular checkups with your doctor are absolutely essential.

The most common cancer in women is of the breast, and 80 percent of all cases occur in women over fifty. According to the American Cancer Society, the rate of breast cancer deaths has doubled in the years 1961–1991. That's why monthly self-exams and yearly mammograms must become a regular part of your life. A mammogram, which is X-rays of different views of your breast tissue—can detect lumps you can't feel, and a few minutes of your time can save your life. Even if you have breast cancer, the five-year survival rate—if the cancer has not spread to the lymph nodes—is an impressive 93 percent. Still, sedentary women are three times more likely to develop breast cancer than active women. Some studies claim that too much fat in your diet can trigger a cancer. And there is a link between levels of the hormone estrogen with breast cancer, as well as genetic links, especially if your mother or sister had it.

This doesn't mean you should panic but that you should take care of yourself and never skip a yearly exam.

You should also have a yearly pelvic exam by your gynecologist. She can feel your organs—uterus and ovaries—to check for any changes in size or shape. A Pap test checks the cells of your cervix.

As you get older you should also have yearly, painless checks for colon cancer. Ask your doctor what is the best for you.

Being overweight also heightens your cancer chances. "When people consume excess calories, it stimulates the metabolic overdrive into making cells divide faster," explains Dr. Daniel Nixon of the American Cancer Society. "This increases the risk that something can go awry, resulting in cancerous cells. Then, too, fat people have more cells, so there is an increased statistical chance that some of these cells might become cancerous."

There are other risk factors for cancer, including certain drugs and your diet. Oral contraceptives and hormone replacement therapy for menopause, for example, lessen your risk of ovarian and endometrial cancer, yet may heighten your risk of breast cancer. Fertility drugs may lead to ovarian cancer. Smoking definitely causes cancer—a recent study by the National Cancer Institute showed a 65.3 percent increase in lung cancer in women in the last decade. So do overexposure to the sun and other environmental factors like pollution and pesticides. You must discuss your options and risk factors with your doctor.

Your diet is also crucial in cancer prevention. An unhealthy diet of fast foods high in sugar, fat, and white flour can lead to colon cancer. The American Cancer Society has issued the following food guidelines to help prevent cancer:

> Maintain a desirable body weight.
>
> Eat a varied diet.
>
> Include a variety of both vegetables and fruit in your daily diet.
>
> Eat more high-fiber foods.
>
> Cut down on fat.
>
> Limit consumption of alcohol.
>
> Limit consumption of salt-cured, smoked, and nitrite-preserved foods.

Call the Cancer Information Service at 1-800-4-CANCER for more information and advice about treatments.

Heart Disease

Heart disease kills more Americans than all other diseases combined, but many of the nearly 500,000 heart attacks in this country could have been prevented. They are most often the result of arteriosclerosis, or hardening of the arteries; in its most common form, called atherosclerosis, there is a gradual buildup of fatty deposits called plaque in your arteries, blocking the blood flow in your body. If the artery leading to your heart is affected, the result is a heart attack; if the arteries leading to your brain are affected, the result is a stroke.

According to the American Heart Association, cigarette smoking, high cholesterol, hypertension (high blood pressure), and not exercising put you at prime risk for heart disease. A diet that's too high in fat, especially saturated fat (see chapter 3), leads to high levels of cholesterol, which clog up your arteries, which cause blood flow to be blocked by plaque. Risk is also determined by excessive and prolonged stress, other diseases, your family gene pool, and your gender, which means women after menopause are especially at risk. "In the 1950s and 1960s, heart disease was considered a normal part of aging," explains Dr. Steven Horowitz, chief of cardiology at the Beth Israel Hospital in Manhattan. "Heart disease among women got overlooked because women tend to develop coronary artery disease in their sixties, a decade later than do men because female hormones protect women until menopause."

You can't change your age, gender, or family predisposition to heart disease, but you can change your diet and lifestyle to greatly reduce your chances of dying from it. That's especially important for us, as we tend to become *less* active as we get older, which is exactly the time when we need to stay *most* active. The buildup of plaque in your arteries can be reversed. Exercise does strengthen your bones, which is especially important for postmenopausal women, to prevent not only osteoporosis but atherosclerosis as well.

Changing diet and lifestyle are not impossible goals. But as with everything else you'll be reading about in this book, changing your body and your attitude is not an overnight process. There's no magic pill alone that will reduce cholesterol if you keep eating too much of it;

there's no instant weight-loss diet that can undo a lifetime of overeating; there's no painless way to stop smoking. Important changes take time. But they will happen, if only you let them.

*Do be aware of what heart attack symptoms can feel like. It's not always sudden chest pain, which often comes out of nowhere and can radiate down your left arm, or into your back and/or jaw. Sometimes a heart attack can be happening when you have pressure in your chest, especially if you get sweaty, heated, or nauseated; or you have a sudden shortness of breath; or even if you feel flooded with a strange feeling of doom. Discuss all these potential symptoms with your doctor. If you think you may be having a heart attack, don't delay. Get immediate help. Insist on being seen by a cardiac specialist and having the necessary tests done. Your life is too valuable to take any chances with a possible heart attack.

Diabetes

Insulin is a hormone made by your pancreas that controls the levels of blood sugar (glucose) in your body. Without insulin, your body cannot metabolize sugars and starches in food to create the energy you need to survive. Type 1 diabetes means your body produces little or no insulin itself, so you need to inject synthetic insulin every day; Type 2 diabetes, which is more common, can often be corrected by changes in your diet, exercise, and oral medication. Exercise improves how your body uses insulin and helps regulate your blood sugar. Changes in diet are crucial. When you eat sugar, you get a burst of quick energy—which quickly disappears. Lots of sugar means lots of insulin, which means overstimulation of the pancreas . . . and as you age, your pancreas has a harder time keeping up with all this stress—especially if you compound this with too much alcohol—and diabetes can be the result. (It's the seventh leading cause of death in America.) A recent study showed that one-pack-a-day smokers are twice as likely as nonsmokers to get adult-onset diabetes.

As diabetics tend to have circulatory problems, especially with their feet, you must work closely with your doctor to find the best diet and exercise plan to keep yourself healthy.

Alzheimer's Disease

You can't find your glasses or remember the name of your neighbor. You're losing your mind—or your memory, you think. Then you panic, certain it's the onset of a dreaded and incurable disease. Alzheimer's can strike anyone, even a former president like Ronald Reagan, and happens most often in people over eighty (one in three). Alzheimer's is caused by a loss of nerve cells, and progressive mental decline—memory loss, disorientation, inability to communicate—and physical deterioration follow. It can be especially heartbreaking for families to watch loved ones slowly seem to lose their very selves.

Much more study and hope is needed. A correct diagnosis is crucial, because other curable diseases have similar symptoms. Caregivers especially need a support network to help them cope.

Prescription Drugs

It's very easy to forget that prescription medications are powerful chemicals with potential side effects. Be a smart consumer, and ask both your pharmacist and your doctor about what a prescription is supposed to do, how a prescription can make you feel, how often you should take it, if you should eat or not eat food with it (some irritate an empty stomach), if it's okay to drink alcohol when on this drug, and how it can interact with any other drugs you're taking and if you should stop taking them. These questions are absolutely crucial, because many drugs not only interact with food but with each other, and can cause very serious problems. You must *always* tell your doctor what other drugs you're taking, whether, for example, hormone-replacement or birth-control pills, over-the-counter cough syrup, or even large doses of vitamins and minerals. Always finish a prescription, even if you feel better right away. Report any unexpected reactions like headaches, dizziness, nausea, and rashes to your doctor immediately. *Never* take more than the prescribed dose.

High Blood Pressure and Strokes

Your blood pressure tends to rise as you age, and each woman has her own "normal" resting figure. If your blood pressure is higher than normal (above 140/90 if you're younger than 60; 160/95 if you're over 60), then you have hypertension—along with 30 percent of all Americans. This puts you at a greater risk for heart attacks, strokes—the third leading cause of death in America—and kidney disease. Most people don't know they have hypertension until it's too late—they have three to four times the risk for heart disease and up to seven times the risk of a stroke. That's why hypertension is often called a Silent Killer.

What causes hypertension? A high-salt diet, alcohol, smoking, obesity, and stress. Hypertension is one ailment that is most often caused by your own behavior.

How can you prevent it? Reduce the sodium in your diet, stop excessive drinking, stop smoking, and lose weight. Learn how to manage stress. One prominent study found that women who ate plenty of fruits and vegetables rich in antioxidant nutrients (see the Vitamin section in chapter 3 for more information on antioxidants) had a 54 percent lower risk of stroke than other women. The choice is up to you.

Menopause and Hormonal Changes

Most of us, so conditioned to think that youth is the only desirable stage of a woman's life, dread the sound of the word *menopause*: the change of life. You're no less a woman because your body stops ovulating and producing the hormones called estrogen and progesterone. Each woman has different symptoms; some start early, at age forty, or late, at age fifty-eight, while others start and stop, and still others don't experience too much distress. For most women menopause begins at around the age of 50 and can continue over a period of up to five years. As estrogen levels drop, we can have hot flashes and perspiration, insomnia, memory lapses, dizziness, trouble breathing, vaginal dryness and lessened libido, heart palpitations as well as get depressed not only by the physical symptoms but the emotional response they bring to all of us. We're also at much higher risk of osteoporosis.

As we learn more about menopause, the buzzwords are *Hormone Replacement Therapy* (HRT). Taking supplements of estrogen and progestin (as creams, pills, injections, or skin patches) will not only alleviate many of the menopause symptoms but can also greatly reduce the risk of both heart disease and uterine cancer. HRT can also reduce the fracture risk from osteoporosis by 5 to 60 percent; decrease the duration and frequency of hot flashes; and improve vaginal lubrication. Unfortunately, HRT might also increase the risk of breast cancer. More studies need to be done, and you must discuss all your options with your doctor; as the benefits of reduced heart disease–risk often far outweigh the cancer risks.

Your doctor must also be very sympathetic to your symptoms and take them seriously. If he or she isn't, then find another doctor—ask your friends for recommendations. There's nothing to be afraid of or embarrassed about. If your doctor tells you a hysterectomy—removal of the uterus, the second most common surgical procedure done on women, and major, painful, often unnecessary surgery—is your only solution, do yourself a favor and get a second or third opinion. There are many alternatives to such radical and overprescribed surgery.

Making changes in your diet as well as developing a regular exercise routine can help alleviate many menopause symptoms, as well as give you an outlet for emotions that may be fluctuating like crazy. If you have trouble sleeping, for instance, try eating a small and early dinner (this will also help prevent fat storage). Eat five minimeals a day to keep those carbohydrates coming in to stabilize your blood sugar levels. Eat nutrient-dense foods to increase your vitamin and mineral levels. Boost your metabolism and endorphins with regular exercise. Alternative therapies like acupuncture, herbs, aromatherapy, and massage can do wonders as well.

I see menopause as a welcome time for you to focus on *your* health and *your* future. It's quite normal to have seesawing emotions and worries; hopefully your loved ones will respond with sympathy and support. Your friends and colleagues and women's support groups can help as well. Don't hesitate to seek out advice, and you'll also find many wonderful books in the women's health section in your local bookstore.

Thyroid Disease

Millions of women have hypothyroidism, or underactive thyroid glands, and suffer years of distress because they are not diagnosed properly. These little glands in your neck pump out the hormones that regulate most of your body functions, and a simple blood test, called a TSH assay, measures the hormone levels. Be sure to ask for one whenever you get a physical.

According to the American Association of Clinical Endocrinologists, these are some of the possible symptoms of hypothyroidism:

Tiredness, loss of interest and/or pleasure, forgetfulness

Dry coarse hair, and loss of outer eyebrow hair

Puffy face and eyes

Slow heartbeat

Intolerance to cold

Heavy or irregular periods (if premenopausal)

Constipation

Goiter (overenlarged thyroid gland)

Dry skin

Weight gain

Brittle nails

Osteoporosis and Arthritis

Osteoporosis

Our bones hold us up and keep us together, and we certainly take them for granted. Most of us assume that once we reach our full height, our bones will never change during our lifetime. In truth, our bones are dynamic, wonderful things that constantly change and remodel themselves, and can actually respond and adjust to the demands placed upon them. Bones need to be used, or they become less dense when mineral salts—mostly calcium—are gradually withdrawn. And when bone density decreases, we are susceptible to osteoporosis and fractures.

Osteoporosis is something you must be aware of—half of all women between the ages of forty-five and seventy-five show some signs of it, and there are over one million osteoporosis fractures each year. It is often called a silent disease because you don't know you have it until a bone breaks, most often in your hip, wrist, or spine. Osteoporosis is caused by several factors: our genes, our gender, and our race, which can't be changed; but it is also caused by the calcium in our diet, how much exercise we do, and our estrogen levels, which we can change. Women are particularly susceptible to osteoporosis, especially when we don't have enough estrogen, a hormone that helps maintain bone density, or calcium in our diets. (Constant low-calorie dieting means we eat fewer of the calcium-rich foods we need. Furthermore, diet sodas and protein contain phosphoric acid, which upsets the necessary ratio of phosphorus to calcium in our bodies, and helps contribute to bone loss.) Calcium is stored in our bones until it's needed for many vital body functions. If you eat too much protein, salt, and caffeine, which stress your kidneys and deplete calcium, and you don't eat enough foods (like low-fat dairy and green leafy vegetables) with calcium, your body will borrow it from your bones, and they weaken. They break. You fall. You hurt. You feel old.

It's up to you to lessen the risk of having osteoporosis ravage your bones. The best way to strengthen bones is by exercising. The best way to put calcium in your body is to eat it in *food*, not in supplements, although few of us actually do that with a healthy, balanced diet. The RDA for calcium is 800 milligrams, but most of us ingest much less. The National Institute of Health recommends that postmenopausal women who aren't taking estrogen supplements have at least 1,500 milligrams of calcium daily.

It's easy to add calcium to your diet. See my suggestions in chapter 3. There are also many kinds of calcium supplements to buy. Discuss with your doctor which is the best kind for you and when you should take them, as they have different rates of absorption in your body.

Arthritis

There are an estimated thirty-seven million Americans with some form of arthritis, and there's no cure for it. Still, we spent upwards of $1 billion in the hope that some unproven remedy is going to help ease the pain. Osteoarthritis, or degenerative wear and tear on the joints, comes with aging. The most common form of arthritis is rheumatoid, which is an inflammation of the membrane surrounding your joints.

Arthritis can involve only one joint or many; be a mild ache or crippling agony. It is treated with antibiotics, anti-inflammatory drugs to bring down swelling, bed rest, an exercise plan, and changes in diet—which means weight loss to take strain off your weary joints. Sadly, many of the drugs have life-threatening side effects, so you must be monitored carefully once on them. Drugs that seem to work for one person may not work for you.

Many women erroneously think that exercise is not good for arthritis, but that's usually not true, unless you're having a flare-up. Once your doctor has said you can exercise, go ahead. Believe me—it can really help. Just go very slowly, as a long, slow, very gradual warm-up is a must. Callanetics can help you tremendously here, because you'll be *working at your own pace*, and *listening to your body*. Working out can improve circulation and range of motion in arthritic joints as well as relieve pain and prevent further deformities.

Skin: Wrinkles and Cancer

Skin is our body's largest organ. It covers and protects every bit of us and reflects all the things—good and bad—we put in our bodies. A healthy diet and lots of water will obviously be reflected in glowing, hydrated skin; poor nutrition, smoking and tanning, and lack of exercise show just as much, if not more. Junk food has empty calories and makes you fat. Salt makes you puffy. Fried food is full of grease—guess where it goes! Too much caffeine and alcohol make you look pasty and drawn out. Who needs it? Not you!

Wrinkles

Oh, those wrinkles, etched into our faces. They're not supposed to be there. We're supposed to be young and unlined and gorgeous forever. Or rather, lines and creases and all the experience of feelings are okay and even look sexy on a man's face (just think of Sean Connery), but women are running to the cosmetic surgeon faster than you can say "face-lift" if they see the slightest hint of a droop.

Our skin naturally loses elasticity and moisture as we age, mainly due to lower levels of estrogen and progesterone, but we certainly don't help it by our thoughtless behavior. Namely: sun worship. Most skin damage is not caused by aging but by overexposure to the sun. The sun's rays *are* harmful. A tan is *not* healthy; it does not prevent wrinkles or age spots—it causes them. Society and magazines telling us we look good when we're tanned are *wrong*. But because, like so many other diseases, skin damage can take years to show upon your face, the damage has already been done. You need only look at Brigitte Bardot's leathery, lined face, to see what summer fun in the sun did to her.

We spend hundreds and hundreds of dollars each year on the newest moisturizers and creams to plump up our faces, yet we don't think to protect ourselves properly when we go out of the house. Two-thirds of skin damage is "incidental," not from a vacation—which means it happens every time you walk out of the house and into the light, no matter where you live or what time of year.

Savvy cosmetics companies are starting to make moisturizers, foundations, and lipsticks with a built-in SPF (Sun Protection Factor), which is a terrific idea. There are also lots of new products containing AHAs, or alpha-hydroxy acids, found in fruits, sugarcane, and sour milk. AHAs are exfoliants, which take off the dead outer layers of skin, refining its texture and rejuvenating the complexion. A qualified dermatologist or skin-care specialist can also do a professional acid peel, where more layers of skin are removed and wrinkles lessened. Do shop around if you decide to have a peel, and be sure to speak up, especially if your skin tends to be easily irritated. It's crucial to find the right person to do a peel, as scarring is a real possibility if it's not done properly. Peels also need to be repeated every few weeks or months for maximum benefit, but it's a lot safer, less drastic, and far less expensive than cosmetic surgery.

I firmly believe in the importance of a simple, consistent skin-care plan. Don't overclean your face and never use hand or deodorant soap on it; it's irritating, drying, and not necessary. Remove all your makeup before going to bed. Always moisturize. Use a humidifier in your house (and especially in the bedroom at night) to keep the air hydrated. Drink lots of water.

Don't believe all the hype at the cosmetics counters. If you find a product you like, stick with it. Just remember that your skin gets drier as you age, so products that might have been adequate a few years ago might not be so effective. Use a light hand when applying makeup, especially with harsh or bright colors, or cakey textures that play up skin imperfections. A little pampering goes a long way.

I'm not going to go on and on with a lecture about what cigarette smoke does to your face. Suffice it to say that nothing's less sexy than those horrid little lines etched around your mouth from years of puckering and puffing.

Skin Cancer

Skin cancer used to be something we never thought about because it was so rare. It's not anymore, especially with the continuing depletion of the ozone layer that protects us from the sun's rays. We need to worry about UVA (Ultraviolet A), which destroys skin elasticity, causing premature aging and contributing to cancer; and UVB (Ultraviolet B), which causes burns and is thought to be the primary cause of skin cancer. An estimated 700,000 people will be diagnosed with skin cancer this year, resulting in more than 9,100 deaths. More than 90 percent are basal cell or squamous cell carcinomas, which have a cure rate of 95 percent if caught and treated early. Worse, one in 90 Americans will develop a malignant melanoma, the deadliest form, which can spread quickly throughout your body.

Sun Protection:

- Everyone needs protection from the sun. Always use a sunscreen or block, not just on your face and neck, but on your hands and legs and other frequently exposed areas as well. Use the correct SPF for your skin type. An SPF 15, for example, means you can stay out in the sun 15 times longer than if you had no protection. An SPF will not stop you from burning if you sweat or rub it off.

- Always apply a sunscreen at least fifteen minutes before going out, so your skin has a chance to absorb it properly.

- Never use a tanning booth. They are not safe, no matter what the people who use them might say.

- Cover your head and neck with hats and scarves. (I drive with gloves that cover my arms.) We so often forget about moisturizing and taking care of the skin on our neck, and it is especially susceptible to burns.

- Always wear a pair of sunglasses that are UVA and UVB safe.

- Stay out of the sun between 10 A.M. and 3 P.M., when it's at its strongest, especially when you're on vacation in a sunnier place than usual.

- Examine all the skin on your body at least once a month. Make a map of your moles, birthmarks, and blemishes.

- If you see any changes in a mole or any other spot on your skin, see a dermatologist immediately.

The ABCDs of Melanoma:

Asymmetry—One half of a mole doesn't match the other half.

Border irregularity—The edges are ragged, notched, or blurred.

Color—The pigmentation is not uniform. Shades of tan, brown, and black are present. Dashes of red, white, and blue add to the mottled appearance.

Diameter—Greater than six millimeters (about the size of a pencil eraser). Any growth of a mole should be of concern.

Stop Smoking Now

Many women say they don't want to stop smoking because they're afraid they'll gain weight. That's the least of your worries if you smoke. About one in every five deaths in America is caused by smoking. That's 400,000 people every year. Smoking more than doubles your risk of heart disease. The American Cancer Society estimates that smoking causes 75 percent of lung cancer found in women, compounded by a 67 percent higher death rate than nonsmokers. It worsens many other medical conditions, depresses your immune system and makes it harder for you to heal. It can cause a much higher risk for heart attack, strokes, and blood clots in women who are taking birth control pills. If that's not enough, a new study that was just written up in the *Journal of the American Medical Association* states that secondhand smoke is much more harmful to nonsmokers than it is to the smokers themselves. That's because smokers have developed natural protection against the toxic substances in cigarettes, while nonsmokers haven't. The researchers claim that damage caused by passive smoke is America's third leading cause of preventable death, after smoking itself and alcohol abuse. Waitresses have the highest cancer rate of any female occupation. According to the Occupational Safety and Health Administration, nearly 47,000 people die each year from heart disease caused by secondhand smoke, and 150,000 others suffer nonfatal heart attacks. Those are shocking figures.

There are over 2,500 chemicals in tobacco and over 4,000 in tobacco smoke. Nicotine, the active substance in cigarettes, is highly addictive and harder to kick, say most, than heroin. Withdrawal symptoms are unpleasant: anxiety, restlessness, irritability, disturbed sleep, inability to concentrate, hunger, and, of course, a desperate craving for nicotine. Luckily, your risk of developing cancers, heart disease, and all the dozens of other illnesses related to smoking start to decline as soon as you stop.

Here are a few of the methods for quitting smoking:

Nicotine gum and patches. Ask your doctor for advice and a prescription.

Hypnosis and/or acupuncture. This can help you relax.

Cold turkey. Easier said than done. It takes tremendous willpower and determination.

Exercise. Start slowly. Once your breathing gets easier, you may find some extra incentive to keep you away from the cigarettes. Fortunately, many former smokers find that some form of exercise does help them kick the habit. Not only do they have more wind and energy, but aerobics helps prevent the weight gain so many women are afraid of and provides a healthy outlet for the stress of nicotine withdrawal.

A support group that might help you quit is Nicotine Anonymous. For a local meeting, send a business-sized, self-addressed, stamped envelope to Nicotine Anonymous World Service, Dept. A, P.O. Box 591777, San Francisco, CA 94159-1777.

You can also call the American Lung Association at 1-800-LUNG-USA for booklets, videos, and information about smoking-cessation clinics near you.

Accepting Your Body: Graceful Aging

Learn to love your body. Each one of us has her own unique shape and body type. Women are meant to have lovely round breasts and round hips. This is a good time to look at your body. Do you like to look at it? Does it drive you crazy? Do your clothes fit? Do you have one set of fat clothes and one set of thin clothes? Do you enjoy sex without having to hide under the sheets? Train yourself to look in the mirror and find what you like about your own body. Even if you're an identical twin, no one else has one exactly like it. The only ideal body is one that is healthy, strong, and flexible. The ideal body will be brimming with energy and vitality, not starved into submission.

It's only human nature to constantly compare ourselves with nearly every other woman we see. Is she thinner? Is she younger? Well, maybe she's thin on top, but she has a gooshy behind, or thunder thighs, or saggy breasts. It's amazing how much rueful comfort we get from putting down other women's bodies to make us feel better about our own perceived deficiencies, isn't it? I learned a valuable lesson once, years before Callanetics transformed my life, when I was in a very classy restaurant in New York, and seated at the next table was an incredibly beautiful, lithe young woman with a gorgeous man. I'll never look like that, I told myself, so perfect and leggy and lean, with that kind of date. Well, after my meal, I went to the ladies room, and there was Miss Leggy, bent over the toilet, throwing up her dinner. The woman I'd been so admiring was bulimic, tortured with an eating disorder to keep that trim figure. Believe me, my envy went flying right out the window. No one should ever have to go through such extremes of self-abuse to be thin.

And how much time do we waste being jealous that our girlfriend can literally seem to eat whatever she wants, and not gain an ounce? The truth is that naturally thin people usually don't overeat. They *listen to their bodies*, and eat what they need, and then stop. Occasionally they eat a piece of chocolate, or a small serving of low-fat frozen yogurt, and then stop. It can really be wonderful to see a person who has healthy eating habits; for them, it's just something you do when you're hungry, with no emotional strings attached.

Plastic surgery is so popular because it seems to promise a quick fix for all our body dissatisfaction. Liposuction, for example, is major surgery to remove fat cells. The problem is, if you (over)eat the same amount of food and sit around instead of exercising, you'll soon fill the remaining fat cells in your body and look the same if not worse as you did before surgery. I have one friend who had liposuction on her thighs and behind and soon grew an enormous belly—it seemed that her fat deposits had shifted. She was going crazy but refused to exercise, because it was too "boring."

A perfect example of graceful aging is a lovely woman named Ruth Jeffries, a fifty-six-year-old divorced mother of four grown children, who runs the Callanetics exercise studio in New York. I'd like her to tell her story here, because she is someone who has completely transformed her body, her attitude about fitness and health, and her life.

"The first time I ever tried Callanetics was over the Fourth of July weekend, when my children were away and all my friends were busy," Ruth explains. "For some reason I picked up the *Callanetics* book—I didn't know there was a video—mainly because it said it would make you ten years younger in ten hours! Well, I spent the entire weekend on the floor, my glasses falling off my face, patient and determined to master the exercises. At one point, doing a hamstring stretch, I suddenly thought, Wow! This is really intense—like a shock to my system. I didn't know what had happened, but it was as if my body were literally trying to tell me it needed these exercises. It made me determined to succeed.

"The more I did Callanetics and the stronger I became, the more I watched my body change shape. I used to travel quite a lot for my old job, and I could do Callanetics in my hotel room, or even take quick breaks in the office. My blood pressure went down to 110/70, and my resting pulse is 52, which is incredibly low. My breasts are higher than they've ever been; my jawline is tighter and I no longer have any double chins; my stomach is flatter; and my behind is lifted higher than it was when I was a teenager. I have improved my nimbleness, reflexes, and reaction time, which is especially important now that I live in New York!

"I became convinced that Callanetics was the right program for aging baby boomers, many of whom had stress-related injuries or gym burnout, and had tried and failed at other exercise routines. I knew it was right for me. I was tired of working in the corporate world and of all the traveling I had to do; it was too stressful and made me feel old. So I decided to buy the New York Callanetics franchise. That way I'd be working for myself, doing something I knew was keeping me young.

"Callanetics allows you to exercise at your own pace, using the power of your own body. Strength and flexibility are the key issues as we get old, and Callanetics helps you improve both. The women who come to this studio are different; they're interested in getting in touch with their own bodies, their own sexuality—let me tell you, pelvic rotations can really help improve your sex life! And they're fed up, as I am, with the media telling us we aren't sexy if we're not twenty-five years old. They're willing to listen, to *work at their own pace*. They keep coming because of the incredibly fast results.

"I see Callanetics as the intelligent woman's exercise. It teaches you to concentrate, which improves your memory. It teaches you patience. It calms you, forcing you to relax. It improves your breathing. It uses every fiber of your body. It has completely changed my body and my life."

Callanetics can work for anyone, no matter what your age or fitness level. It is only because we have gone to the extremes of no exercise and excessive food intake that our bottoms have spread and a healthy, natural weight seems an impossible goal. A consistent exercise program, four to five days a week, for only thirty to sixty minutes is all the time you need to become physically fit. Moderate amounts of fat and calories will quickly reestablish a healthy energy balance. You don't have to run a marathon or deprive yourself of your favorite foods to become naturally thin and fit. Callanetics will help you do it.

CHAPTER

STRENGTHEN YOUR HEART

Everyone can benefit from some type of exercise. It doesn't matter how old, how unfit, how overweight or underweight, how coordinated or experienced you are.

I once was traveling and started talking to a couple who were the perfect picture of health: about seventy-five years old, with lean bodies, clear, sparkling eyes, and rosy cheeks. I asked them what kind of exercise they did, and they told me they didn't do any. But how, I wondered, could they be in such outstanding condition without any exercise? Finally they admitted that they walk five miles every day—but they didn't consider that to be exercise, because they enjoyed it so much.

Every step forward counts. The more you do, the more you can do. Aging is not a disease. In fact many of the physical changes we blame on "aging" are a direct result of inactivity. Physical discomfort seemed inevitable because we rarely exercised—certainly not as we got older. That perception has changed. It's no longer considered dangerous for even the very elderly to improve their strength greatly with exercise.

You don't have to win a race to be physically fit. Your fitness level is not measured by your speed or how big your muscles are but by the soundness of your cardiovascular system, how *strong* your muscles are, how flexible you are, and how much body fat you have.

Nor do you need to exercise every day to reap the benefits. Here's what exercise can do for you:

- Lower your risk for nearly every disease, from colds to cancer
- Strengthen your heart and lungs
- Lower your blood pressure
- Keep your weight down
- Maintain and even increase bone density
- Strengthen your immune system
- Lower the percentage of body fat
- Increase the "good" HDL cholesterol and decrease the "bad" LDL cholesterol
- Relieve stress and tension
- Reduce the chances of lower-back problems
- Change the shape of your body
- Increase your range of motion
- Improve reflexes, memory, and coordination
- Improve your sex life
- Stimulate the release of endorphins, which give your body a natural "high" feeling of euphoria
- Relieve depression
- Change your self-image and self-esteem
- Lengthen your life

What Do I Need to Do?

There is no such thing as a short-term commitment to exercise. Exercising is a lifetime commitment to becoming and staying fit. It's the same as a diet plan—there are short-term "quick fixes" that never last and can hurt you. Slow and steady will win the race every time. *Listen to your body.*

The best way to look at exercise is: Train to Gain, Not to Maintain. This means always having a goal. It can be to run a mile or be able to walk up the stairs without wheezing. Once you've attained that goal, you'll set a new one, and always work toward that new one. If you only work out to maintain, then I see it as the same as going backwards. As with anything worthwhile, setting our sights on something concrete keeps us thinking, engaged in the task, and focused. We get stimulated, mentally and physically. We don't get bored. We feel alive and worthwhile. We are pleased with our progress. It's what life is all about, isn't it?

Think of a balanced exercise program as a pyramid with three sections, similar to the food pyramid. At the base is *Cardiovascular Aerobic Exercise*—the strengthening of your heart and lungs. This is the most important support of any exercise program. Aerobic means "with oxygen," which is what is provided for the muscles you work when you are using your body for at least twenty minutes without stopping. (It takes that long for your body to get it together—no one ever said it would be easy!) Aerobic exercise burns fat because it is a readily available source of energy. This is where CardioCallanetics will come in.

Next come *Flexibility Exercises* to improve your range of motion and circulation. Stretching helps keep joints lubricated, which helps prevents stiffness. Moves are performed slowly and carefully to encourage muscles to relax and lengthen. As with any exercise, it is crucial to learn how to stretch properly to avoid injuries.

At the top are *Muscular Endurance* and *Muscular Strength*. Exercises to improve your muscles create resistance against them to teach them how to contract more efficiently, so they become stronger and more toned. Callanetics give you deep muscle tone from very specific movements—without the use of weights or any other equipment.

Callanetics combines strengthening with flexibility. Your muscles must be both relaxed and warmed up to stretch properly, which is why my exercises are so safe to do. When you do Callanetics, you learn to focus on isolating and then relaxing the muscles or groups of muscles that should be working or stretching during each exercise. This superior isolation is what makes Callanetics unique and so effective.

Remember, improving your muscle tone and mass—strengthening and increasing the amount of muscle you have—will increase your metabolic rate and improve your vitality as well as decrease your appetite. So get ready to get moving today!

How Much Exercise Do I Need?

You don't have to exercise every day to reap the many benefits of physical activity. Moderate exercise will improve your overall health and vitality.

If Your Goal Is	Aerobic Exercise*	CardioCallanetics
General Fitness or Maintenance	3 times/week for at least 20 consecutive minutes	2 times/week for at least 30 minutes
Fat Loss	4–5 times/week for approximately 30 minutes	3 times/week for 30–60 minutes
Increased Muscle Tone	3 times/week for at least 20 minutes	2 times/week for 30–60 minutes

*This time refers to exercising at your Target Heart Rate and does not include warm-ups or cooldowns, which are a must. Be sure to budget at least five to ten minutes of warm-ups and cooldowns with each CardioCallanetics session. (Prepared with the assistance of Ellen M. Laura)

- The lovely thing about Callanetics is that it combines strength training with flexibility. For the average adult, two to three strength sessions a week are enough.
- If you do some form of aerobic exercise three times a week, for at least twenty *consecutive* minutes within a target heart range, then you'll be getting cardiovascular benefits.
- If your goal is to lose weight, you may need to work out aerobically between thirty to sixty minutes each time. Work up to three twenty-minute sessions per week, and try this for two weeks. If you're not losing any weight, gradually add time to your workouts, but no more than 10 percent a week. The exact amount of exercise you need to lose weight depends on your body type and your metabolic rate.

Fat burning, unfortunately, is not all that simple. First, fat burning is a learned activity. Muscle cells must learn how to burn fat, and then fat cells must learn how to release fat to muscle cells. This doesn't happen overnight; usually from about three months to a year of consistent aerobic exercise are required. (That's one reason it's so easy to get frustrated and give up.)

Second, for the fat-burning process to occur, the exercise must, as I've said, continue for at least 20 minutes. Moderate intensity is the best. (High-intensity activities burn more calories, but not necessarily *fat* calories.)

Third, you need blood sugar (and I don't mean a candy bar). Look at it this way: Imagine that burning fat is like burning a log. If you light a match and hold it to the log, what happens? The match goes out—because what you need is kindling. In our bodies, sugar is the kindling for burning fat. No blood sugar, no fat burning. Complex carbohydrates like fruit or a whole-wheat bagel or a plain baked potato are the best foods to supply blood sugar for exercise (see chapter 3).

Fourth, the exercise intensity—how hard you work—must force your heart rate up to what's called a Target Heart Range (see below). When we exercise very slowly, our heart doesn't need to work any harder than normal, and it can't get any stronger. When we do too much, our heart poops out and so do we. But when we find the perfect, *moderate* heart rate, which is between 60 to 85 percent of our maximum heart rate, we use oxygen, burn fat, and improve cardiovascular conditioning. Don't forget that your heart is a muscle!

How to Find Your Target Heart Rate (THR)

When I talk about heart rate, all it means is how many beats per minute. You can take your pulse when you're exercising by finding the right spot on your wrist, temple, or your neck. You only need to count the heartbeats for ten seconds and multiply that by six (sixty seconds in a minute). If your math is as bad as mine is you can also take your pulse for six seconds and add a zero to it. For example, if, after six seconds, your pulse is fourteen, add a zero = 140. *Voila!*

To find your THR: Subtract your age from 220. This will give you an estimate of your Maximum Heart Rate (MHR). Your Target Heart Rate (THR) is between 60 to 85 percent of your MHR.

Let's say you're forty-five.

MHR:	$220 - 45 = 175$
60 percent of your MHR:	$175 \times .60 = 105$
80 percent of your MHR:	$175 \times .85 = 148.75$

Your THR is between 105 and 148 beats per minute

What CardioCallanetics Can Do for You

CardioCallanetics is an incredible new, innovative way to strengthen your heart and lungs. What it does is use concepts from ballet and yoga in fluid, graceful patterns that keep you moving continuously for thirty minutes of cardiovascular exercise. But you don't have to worry that it's anything like traditional low-impact aerobics! Those classes use music at 140 to 155 beats per minute—way too fast for most of us. CardioCallanetics works at 110 to 118 beats per minute. You get a maximum workout with a minimum of stress.

A typical CardioCallanetics program consists of a ten-minute warm-up and stretch section, followed by a twenty-minute workout section, and then a half hour of regular Callanetics. The movements are all flowing, slow, and controlled, so they're easy to keep doing. You'll be warmed up so you won't have to worry about injuries, and you'll be using a full range of motion, which means you use more muscle and burn more calories.

Compared to a traditional low-impact aerobic session, CardioCallanetics has a much lower impact on your body. As you know from reading about osteoporosis, impact is not necessarily a bad thing. It increases bone density, strengthens tendons and ligaments, and makes your muscles more resilient. This helps improve posture and prevent osteoporosis. But you still have to be careful. Your workout should challenge your body without being overly stressful to your bones and joints.

All of us need both muscle strength and endurance for optimal health. As you know, Callanetics tones and strengths your body. The Cardio portion of CardioCallanetics increases your body's endurance. If you only increase your endurance, your strength will not necessarily be increased. (This is why so many runners may be fit and have strong legs but have a very untoned upper body.) If you increase your strength, however, you *will* increase your endurance. That's why traditional Callanetics is a must; it makes and keeps you strong—and lets you quickly adapt to CardioCallanetics.

For all about the CardioCallanetics program, please read chapter 6.

Getting Started

Everyone has to start somewhere.

I've heard every kind of excuse from people about why they can't exercise. I have a bad back. I have bad knees. My mother told me not to because I have asthma. My husband says it'll make my legs too big and bulky. I'm totally uncoordinated. I don't feel like it. It's boring. The shoes are ugly.

Let me tell you about Amanda, whom I met when she was nearly eighty pounds overweight. Slowly, she began to eat more healthy food, took daily walks, and went to a support group. After a few weeks she happily reported two experiences that proved to her how quickly her fitness level was changing. First of all, she was able to reach down to her feet and tie her shoes, something we all take for granted but a simple, necessary gesture she'd been unable to do for years because of the fat around her middle. The second event was being able to walk easily all the way up a long flight of stairs at a stadium when she went to root for her hometown baseball team. She used to have to rest at least four or five times on her way up. These were major achievements for her, and her pleasure in her accomplishments helped keep her going. She soon started Callanetics classes and has transformed her body—and her self-image.

You can *learn* to be active. This means you take the stairs instead of the elevator. This means you park your car a block away from where you have to be, or at the far end of a parking lot and walk a little bit farther than you did the day before. This means you get up and walk around when you're talking on the telephone. This means you mow the lawn with an old-fashioned powerless mower, or you rake the leaves in the fall with a rake and not a leaf blower, that you till the soil in your garden by yourself.

The more active we are, the more calories we burn.

The more passive we are, the more exhausted we become . . . and the more unlikely we are to exercise.

When people make a healthy decision for themselves and decide to work out, they often make several (understandable) mistakes that not only diminish their exercise pleasure, but lead them to quit. It's not a simple task to find the time or the motivation. It can be a lonely, disheartening experience if you're not sure what you're doing. It's so easy to get discouraged, especially if you're short of breath.

Others throw themselves into a frenzy of working out and try to do too much too soon, risking injuries. And then all that eager energy will soon be replaced with frustration and disappointment.

Start slowly. Always warm up slowly, and then cool down for stretches after every workout session. (Most people don't and wonder why they're always stiff and sore.) If you incorporate these few minutes into your total workout time from the very beginning, you'll have no problem maintaining this as a healthy habit and will be much less stiff and sore. (A little stiffness is normal, especially at first, as your newly strengthening muscles get used to being used!) Picture your muscles as if they were an old rubber band: when we try to stretch it, it barely bends; but if we pull too hard, it breaks. Be gentle!

Refuse to be frustrated. It's very hard not to want to be striding easily instead of huffing and puffing—but stick with it, and you'll get there. It's impossible *not* to improve if you keep going. Be proud of every effort, even if it's only a few minutes each day, and stop comparing yourself to someone else who may have lost more weight and gotten thinner thighs in the same amount of time. Every day spent exercising is another spent making your body healthier and stronger.

Vary your routine. If you do the same exercise routine day in and day out, your muscles will quickly get used to it, and your mind will get used to it too—by being bored. *Diversify* your exercises as much as you can. This can be as simple as changing the path of your walking route, or choosing to do one Callanetics exercise instead of another. It's much easier to keep going when you know you'll be doing something different.

Risk of Injury

You can do Callanetics every day. You can stretch every day. As I've said, you must consult your doctor before starting any exercise program. This means a complete physical checkup; blood tests to check your nutrition, cholesterol, and thyroid levels; and perhaps a stress test to evaluate your cardiovascular system.

If you feel uncomfortable when you're working out, *stop!* If your heart is thumping erratically, or you're unusually short of breath, *stop!* Don't let anyone tell you that pain is good. It's not. Pain is your body's way of telling you that something may be wrong. *Listen to your body!*

If exercising hurts, there's something wrong with either what you're doing, how you're doing it, or the intensity. Be sure you're wearing appropriate clothing, in layers, so you don't overheat or get chilled when you sweat. You're probably doing too much if you feel faint, dizzy, or nauseated when you're working out; if you're unusually sleepy after exercise or slower than usual to get out of bed in the morning; or if you feel achy and awful and sore for days afterward. Many people try to go back to the level where they were after they've had a bad cold or the flu, for example, and come home exhausted and miserable. Or injured. Pace yourself—go slowly. After all, tomorrow is another workout day. *Never compare yourself with anyone else.*

It's not a good idea to exercise on either an empty or full stomach. If you like to exercise when you first get up, eat half a bagel or a piece of toast at least twenty minutes before you start moving. Try not to work out for at least one to two hours after meals, so your food has a chance to digest properly. Otherwise you may get a stomachache and a less efficient exercise session.

If you have an old injury that you're afraid will "act up" if you exercise, think of the alternative. If you remain inactive, the injury will almost certainly get worse as your muscles and bones deteriorate from lack of use. Sometimes this means finding an alternative if the sport you love caused the injury in the first place—like overstressing your knees jogging or developing tennis elbow. Once you've built up your strength and gotten the go-ahead from your doctor, you very well may be able to ease back into your favorite activity.

If you're recuperating from an injury or surgery and have been told to ease back into exercise at a very cautious pace, then be content even if you can only do five minutes at first. Try five minutes the next time, and if you feel okay, go up to five minutes and thirty seconds. Rest for a few hours and then try again. Never keep doing any activity if it's painful. If you're out of condition, you may feel tired, feel out of breath, or have sore muscles and joints. Go slowly. Walk for a few minutes in the morning. Try again before lunch. Try again before dinner. See how you feel. Gradually your endurance will increase and you'll feel better than ever.

SOME EXERCISE MYTHS DISPELLED

I've been thin all my life, so why do I need to exercise?
Just because you're naturally thin doesn't mean you're fit. Next time you see a parade of models on the runway, look carefully. They may be ultraskinny, but a surprisingly large number are flabby, with gooshy, hanging behinds. Not very attractive. And not very healthy, either. Everyone needs to exercise, no matter what her body type. Couch potatoes, even thin ones, are more than three times more likely to die from heart disease and cancer than people who are moderately fit.

Will eating sugar before I work out give me an extra burst of energy?
No. In fact, it'll probably make your workout harder and make you feel worse. When you eat sugar, it quickly goes into your bloodstream and stimulates insulin—a quick rush. And then it goes down just as quickly, making you feel tired and weak. The best thing to eat for sustained energy is some form of complex carbohydrate—an apple or half a bagel—no more than two hours before your workout.

Is a quick, hard workout better than a long, slow one?
No, it's counterproductive. Your goal is to burn fat. When you exercise strenuously, yes, you'll burn more calories, but they'll be from the accessible carbohydrates in your body and not from fat. Slow and steady wins this race.

If I exercise like a maniac, will I get superfit right away?
No, you'll probably get hurt. The most common mistake is trying to do too much too soon. This is when injuries happen and frustration follows. It's too tempting to give up when you've twisted an ankle or pulled a muscle. You must start out slowly, and when the level you're at seems too easy, then take it up a notch. If you're walking, then all this means is walking a little faster. That way your workout doesn't take more time but is more efficient.

If I do too much strength training, will my muscles become bulging and bulky like a male bodybuilder's?
Definitely the opposite with Callanetics—only with very intensive months of training, combined

with special diets and supplements (and probably a whopping dose of potentially fatal steroid drugs), will any woman bulk up like a man.

If it's hot out, is it safe to exercise?
Yes, but you must always hydrate yourself by drinking lots of water before, *during*, and after exercise. The human body has a wonderfully efficient way of acclimating to heat, as long as you exercise regularly. As temperatures gradually rise, your sweating mechanism becomes more proficient. Of course it's always best to exercise early in the day or at dusk, when temperatures are cooling. Try not to exercise outside on days when pollution is terrible or it's warmer than 80 to 90 degrees, or you could put yourself at risk for dehydration and heat stroke.

If I exercise all the time, can I eat whatever I want?
Sorry. Even if your exercise session was fat burning, eating two doughnuts and a pint of ice cream afterwards is still going to put that new fat right back into your bloodstream and then on your behind. (Information courtesy of Ellen M. Laura, from *The Most Fattening Thing You Can Do Is Go on a Diet.*)

Walk Along with Me

Anyone can walk, in a park, on city streets, around a track, inside a mall. You can walk anywhere, anytime, for free. Walking is the only exercise Americans *don't* stop doing when they get older. It's not for sissies, either—walking burns approximately the same amount of calories per mile as jogging does. (The only difference is that jogging does it faster, but with more stress on your joints from the pounding, so it's easier to get injured.) If you walk at a faster pace you won't necessarily burn more calories, but you *will* improve your cardiovascular conditioning. And at any pace, you'll rev up your body's metabolism, and it stays higher even for some time after you've finished your walk.

I've always found it easy to bliss out while walking, whether listening to tapes of words or music, or just savoring my surroundings, or talking with friends. My preferred walking workout goes like this:

• Start with a few minutes of slow walking to warm up your muscles.

• Gradually increase your pace.

- Walk briskly for the bulk of your workout. Take bold strides. Your breathing and speed will increase. Remember, an exercise walk is not a stroll. You'll be moving with determination at a steady pace. Your arms should move freely at your sides—but don't swing them too much. Breathe deeply.

- Gradually slow for a cooldown walk.

- Always stretch for a walk.

  A few tips for walkers:

- Always see your doctor before starting an exercise regime.

- Proper shoes are essential. This means workout shoes made for walking, not running, tennis, or other sports. Good walking shoes give you the right cushioning and support for an upright stride, and help prevent leg strain. Always try on shoes with the kind of athletic socks you wear; I've found it's better to try them on at the end of the day, when your feet have already swollen from a day's use. This will give you a truer fit. Be sure to buy a pair that is snug yet comfortable; you'll want to try on at least three or four pairs before making a decision.

- Wear comfortable clothing. Layers are best. This is especially important if you're walking outside in fluctuating temperatures and wind chills— you can peel down or add on as you warm up or get cooler. There are some marvelous synthetic (and inexpensive) fabrics in workout gear now that "wick" moisture away from your body and keep you comfortable, so you never have to find yourself chilled. Avoid exercising when it's very hot or very cold or very windy. Don't forget a hat and gloves in cold weather, and sunglasses on bright days. Put sunscreen on your face!

- Start slowly and gradually build up endurance. Too much too soon means you're likely to burn out and give up, or get hurt. *Always work at your own pace.* Try starting with twenty minutes several days a week for a month, or until you feel comfortable, and then go up to thirty minutes each time. Try to work up to three miles in forty-five minutes—a fifteen-minute mile—if you can. Take your time getting there. Train to Gain, Not Maintain. A goal is so important!

- Move smoothly. Don't paddle or flap your arms—this wastes energy trying to keep your body in line. Feel your muscles warm as you walk.

Enjoy the day, the swing of your arms, the comfortable speed you've established.

- Carry yourself proudly. Be aware of your posture—your head held high, your chest lifted, shoulders relaxed so you can breathe deeply. Curl your pelvis up as you walk; this will stretch your spine and allow you to feel the contraction in your stomach. Feel your body lift two inches higher. Hold your shoulders up and back. Very soon your body will feel as light as a feather.

- Have fun! Smile...relax...breathe deeply, and don't clench your teeth. Take a Talk Test: If you're so out of breath that you can't talk, you're doing too much. Slow down. If you can talk in your normal voice, you're not working hard enough. Speed it up gradually. Don't worry, as the weeks go by you'll be amazed how quickly your endurance improves and your strength increases.

- The beauty of walking is you set the pace. You do what feels comfortable for you. No one is judging you. Walk tall and think about how good you're being to your body and yourself.

- Always do your stretches (see part 2 for Callanetics stretches) after a walk. This improves flexibility, so all your movements will be fluid and more natural. The best time to stretch is always *after* exercise, when your muscles are warmed up, or after a warm bath. You can even do Callanetics stretches when you're standing in line at the supermarket—your muscles are warmed up from walking around, pushing that cart—or when you're fixing dinner, or even at your desk. Always pay more attention to how you feel when you stretch than how far you can go.

- Don't forget—walking is an aerobic activity, but it only works your lower body. You still should be doing your Callanetics exercises to keep your body stretched and toned. Otherwise you'll get stiff and inflexible, with a sore back. Your stomach exercises are especially important when you become a walker.

- If it's feasible, think about getting a dog. Not only will you have a companion for your walks—and believe me, a dog *needs* to be walked!—but you'll have a loving animal to enrich your life.

Swimming and More

Nonimpact and *low-impact* exercise are confusing terms. Walking is low-impact exercise, because you are exerting about 1.2 times your body weight on your feet and joints with every step. Nonimpact exercise means you're not putting any excess pressure on your body, such as during Callanetics or when you're swimming, because the buoyancy of the water supports your body.

Impact, as I've already told you, is not necessarily such a bad thing, especially when you're healthy. In fact, it's an important ingredient to help strengthen and maintain strong, dense bones. Remember, your bones are miraculously able to adapt to the stresses put on them, and low-impact exercise is one of these stresses.

If you have knee or back problems, swimming, in addition to Callanetics, may be the answer. Not only is it extra-easy on your muscles and bones, but it helps your heart and lungs, your flexibility, your energy, and your state of mind. It's particularly good for overweight women, who will naturally be more buoyant, and won't have to worry about the excess weight slowing them down on the treadmill at the gym.

You may find it easier to work out with exercise classes in the water. These are usually called Aqua Aerobics and can be fun. You have the benefits of exercising in the water with other people, which may be nice if you don't like swimming laps.

Unfortunately, many people do not live near or have access to pools, don't actually like swimming, and feel that having wet hair in the winter is rather annoying!

An alternative nonimpact exercise is dancing. Not only is it aerobic, but it's quite a lot of fun. I love ballroom dancing. The music is lovely, you have a partner working with you, and hours can fly by before you know it. What better way to combine pleasure with exercising?

Other low-impact exercises that are fun and good for you are: bike riding, cross-country skiing, hiking, race walking, even in-line skating!

Taking Care of Your Body as You Exercise

Do you ever start any fitness program without the go-ahead from your doctor. Special precautions must be taken if you're on medication, and you must monitor your heart rate if you have any underlying condition or are taking any drugs for hypertension or any other circulatory problems.

Once the okay is given, here are a few more hints to make your indoor and outdoor workouts more comfortable.

1. Work at your own pace.
2. For Callanetics' sitting and standing exercises, a mat can cushion your feet and bottom.
3. If it bothers you to raise your arms over your head during CardioCallanetics, raise them only as high as is comfortable.
4. Drink lots of water before and after CardioCallanetics exercises.
5. Allow time for an extended cooldown period, of at least ten to fifteen minutes. As we age our heart rate fluctuates, and for some people it sometimes stays higher a little longer than the average. It's perfectly normal, but a long, slow cooldown will ease you back down to your regular heart rate with absolutely no stress.

Remember, nothing in the universe stays at peak performance level at all times, and that includes our bodies. We all have cycles, highs and lows, ups and downs. We need to strive to work at our peak to maintain the high performance levels to keep us from feeling too blue.

As I said, you'll be training to gain, not to maintain. If you find it hard to keep motivated, try keeping an exercise diary, like your food diary and your stress diary. Buy yourself a beautiful bound blank book. Write down every single bit of exercise you do each day. Even if you only manage five minutes of walking, you can still make an entry. The more you do, the quicker your diary will fill up. You'll be amazed at your progress and determination, so if you're having a bad day, just looking at all you've already accomplished can give you a huge boost.

EATING HEALTHY

Why Diets Don't Work

Diets don't work. I've been saying that for the last twenty years because it's true. Just thinking about dieting automatically makes most of us feel deprived. Even the word *diet* misleads us into believing that eating high-quality, delicious, and naturally low-fat foods is a temporary activity, rather than the way we're supposed to be eating all the time. What you can learn to do is rethink the way you eat, learn what it is your body needs, and satisfy its true hunger.

According to the Calorie Control Council, however, forty-eight million adult Americans are dieting. Thirty-one million of these adults are women. Studies have shown that as much as two-thirds of the weight lost through dieting is regained within one year, and nearly all the weight is regained within five years. We're only supposed to be getting 20 to 30 percent of our calories from fat, yet the typical American eats nearly double that. We eat far too much sugar, sodium (salt), and fat, especially saturated fat. We don't eat enough complex carbohydrates. That's why only 15 percent of adults aged forty to forty-nine fall within the recommended weight range.

The first weight you're going to lose is the excess baggage of a dieter's mentality. Many of us don't eat because our bodies tell us they're "hungry" and need fuel to keep going. We eat because we're unhappy, bored, frustrated . . . because it tastes good . . . because we're so used to it we don't know where to begin to stop . . . because it gives us (at least temporarily) some form of comfort and stress reduction.

Eating is a complex and emotionally loaded issue, tied into childhood feelings of nurturing and dependence. Do you eat to satisfy an unmet emotional need? Does it make you feel better when you're stressed and anxious? Are you nutritionally "empty" because you've eaten such poor-quality food? You deserve to eat the best foods to fuel your body and satisfy your hunger, don't you?

Food is often used to control behavior, as a punishment or reward. We learn how food "should" taste from our families. If we grew up in a house that put butter on everything before even tasting it, it's hard to eat an ear of corn that's *not* dripping in butter. But you can retrain your tastebuds to "like" healthier foods, just as you can train your body to do Callanetics.

On top of the emotional issues, finding truly healthy foods is a challenge, especially when we simply don't have time to cook or even think about cooking. Our bodies need more than forty different nutrients for optimal health, and no one single food supplies them all. It's impossible to control the calories of food we don't prepare ourselves. And when we're hungry or bored or exhausted, practically every commercial seems to be for some lusciously fattening calorie-laden yummie. Remember, advertisers are in the business of selling products, not in the business of trying to keep you healthy.

What I'd like to see you do is pay as much attention to your nourishment as you would to a newborn infant. Women aim to give a baby the best-quality food available, breast milk or specially balanced formula to help it grow healthy and strong. No sane woman would give her baby milk it cannot digest. And they also give their babies love and a peaceful, comforting environment while they eat.

This is exactly what we should be doing for ourselves. Successfully thin people may have as many unmet emotional needs as overweight people. The difference is that they don't use food to satisfy feelings of loneliness, anxiety, or boredom.

There is no such thing as a "bad" food: our favorite foods aren't bad in small doses. It's the amount we eat of them that's the problem. Once you learn to stop depriving yourself of what you think is "bad," you'll no longer be so sorely tempted to binge or constantly eat foods that aren't so healthy.

Stop Yo-Yo Dieting Now

Yo-yo dieting is what happens when we lose weight and then gain it all back (and then some). There's a lot of misinformation out there about the hazards of yo-yo dieting, with some studies claiming that a yo-yoing *permanently* slows down your metabolism, or puts you at greater risk for a heart attack and other stressful effects on your body, mainly caused because rapid weight changes may raise blood pressure and cholesterol levels. Other studies conclude that yo-yoing is not in itself terribly harmful to your heart. Everyone at least can agree that even a small weight loss can drastically improve your health. What I believe is that constant weight fluctuations—where you might have a closetful of "fat" clothes and "thin" clothes—are certainly damaging to your state of mind.

The reason yo-yo dieting is such a problem is that when we go on very restrictive diets, we lose both fat and muscle at the same time, but when we start eating again, our metabolism has *temporarily* slowed down, and we regain more fat than muscle. We're also usually so hungry for "bad" foods we've been deprived of that we binge and overeat. So with each successive yo-yo, you put on more and more fat (and get more and more frustrated, making it easier to just give up). In other words: Fast weight loss = water and muscle loss. Whereas: Slow weight loss = fat loss.

The solution to banish the yo-yo diet forever is to change your eating patterns forever. Stop depriving yourself and learn how to eat healthy foods that fill you up for all the right reasons. (Information courtesy of Ellen M. Laura, *The Most Fattening Thing You Can Do Is Go on a Diet.*)

Calories, Diets, and Metabolism

With all this talk about dieting, few of us actually understand what that means, and how our bodies work. A calorie is not your enemy. It is simply a unit of energy. Food contains energy that can be burned or stored, and this energy is measured in calories. If there are no calories in something we eat, it can never give us energy. We also burn energy just by being alive, whether sleeping or exercising, and this energy, too, can be measured in calories. The amount of energy we store depends on how much we take in and how much we burn. If we take in more energy than we burn, we gain weight. If we burn more energy than we take in, we lose weight. Since there are 3,500 calories in one pound of fat, you need a deficit of 3,500 calories to burn off one pound.

That sounds like a lot of calories. The average woman burns between 1,500 to 2,000 calories each day, depending on how active she is. If we cut our food intake to less than 1,200 calories, we'll be burning up muscle along with the fat, and that's the last thing we want. (Remember, developed muscle is what keeps your metabolism high.) We can increase our exercise calories, too, but even a vigorous workout will burn only 500 calories in an hour.

The best strategy is to do a little of both: Cut down on your food calories *and* increase your exercise/activity calories. If all you do is cut back 250 food calories (two handfuls of potato chips, or one candy bar) and add 250 fat-burning calories of exercise (forty-five minutes of a brisk walk), you'll lose a pound a week. Double this to 500 calories and you'll lose two pounds.

And you'll keep it off.

Sounds slow and frustrating, right?

Wrong. If you lose two pounds each week, at the end of month you'll have lost eight pounds. And then forty-eight pounds in six months . . . ninety-six pounds in a year! How much fat do you really need to lose? Let's say the weight's been creeping up over the last ten years. How on earth can ten years of fat melt away overnight? The whole concept of instant weight loss is ridiculous. It takes you at least twelve years to go to school as a child, and then it takes an additional four years to graduate from college—because learning is a slow and meticulous process—and it takes a body awhile to adjust to healthier eating patterns. Fortunately that isn't a four-year process. You *can* lose ten years of thirty to fifty pounds of stored-up excess weight in less than six months. Believe me, that's amazingly fast considering how long that fat took to be stored in the first place.

Think of losing weight as something to be done in Triple Slow Motion. We always think we want everything done right this very minute.

But when it comes to losing fat, fast is not better. In fact, it's not even possible. It takes time for fat cells to learn how to release fat, and then it takes time to burn fat off. You'll learn how effective Callanetics exercises are when done in Triple Slow Motion. The same principle applies to weight loss and management. Slow and steady always wins the race.

Keeping a Food Diary

The *New England Journal of Medicine* reported that the more women diet, the less aware they are of what they're actually eating. Food diaries are tremendously useful tools to pinpoint not only what you eat, but how, when, and *why* you eat what you do. Keep a food diary for a week before you start any new eating plan, and you'll be loading up with so much helpful information that any changes in your eating habits will become much easier. Don't feel embarrssed and certainly don't cheat. This is a tool to help you become fully aware of what you are eating. No one's going to see this except you (and your doctor or nutritionist, if you're getting expert advice). No one is judging you. Here's how to do it:

Take a blank notebook or sheets of paper, and for each day mark off sections for breakfast, lunch, dinner, and snacks. Within these sections mark off:

Food Diary

	Breakfast	Lunch	Dinner	Snacks
Day:				
Food:				
quantity:				
calories:				
fat grams:				
Drinks:				
quantity:				
calories:				
fat grams:				
Total calories:				
Total fat grams:				

	Breakfast	Lunch	Dinner	Snacks
Time begun:				
Time stopped:				
Where I'm eating:				
With whom:				
How this food makes me feel:				

Let's say you have one small glass of orange juice, two scrambled eggs with one tablespoon of butter, two slices of white toast with one tea-spoon of butter and one tablespoon of jam, three cups of coffee with one-half cup of whole milk and three teaspoons of sugar, and a cookie. Look at the labels on all the containers. Write down the calories, portion size, and fat grams if you can. Be sure to add what the food's been cooked in—you'll have to factor in calories from fat used in frying or sautéing, or hidden in sauces or ketchup or salad dressing. Don't forget to write down what you're drinking. Write down exactly what time it is, where you are, and whom you're with. Then write down what you're feeling. Are you hurried, anxious, bored, unhappy, or filled with plea-sure? Do you feel bloated or just plain icky? Then write down how long it took you to eat. Do the same thing for all lunches, dinners, and snacks. Write exact amounts. If you have a salad, don't forget to put down exactly how much dressing you're adding. (This is a good time to start teaching yourself about portion size.)

After a week, you'll have identified not only your eating patterns, but also your patterns of behavior, foods you might have sensitivities to, and what foods are lacking in your diet. You'll see if you eat faster when you're gulping down your breakfast before you rush off to work or sitting at your desk; if eating dairy products makes you bloated and uncomfort-able; how few vegetables you actually eat; how a candy bar in the after-noon makes you feel great for ten minutes and then sluggish and awful an hour later; whether dinner with your family is leisurely and relaxed, so you eat slowly as you unwind . . . and so forth. You'll see how many hidden, extra calories come from liquids. If, for example, you add cream and two sugars to your coffee, that's about 100 calories. Drink four or five cups and you'll have more calories than you probably ate for breakfast. "Natural" sodas still have about 100 calories, as does presweetened iced tea. Everything adds up!

Most important, an accurate food diary will let you know exactly how many calories and fat grams you're eating.

Labels and Learning How to Measure Your Food

Your stomach is about the size of your fist—before you put food into it, that is. If you've already digested all the food from your most recent meal, your stomach would be close to empty. So how much food does it take to fill it up?

A fistful. That's not very much, is it?

Your food diary will tell you *what* you're actually eating and drinking, while food labels and measuring will tell you *how much*. We grossly underestimate the amount of food and calories we eat, because we're just not familiar with what portion sizes are supposed to be. Every time we eat out, restaurants—who want you to come back, remember—load humongous portions on our plates, so we tend to feel gypped if we don't see these vast quantities of food. Once you start measuring the serving sizes you'll see on labels, those portions are shockingly small.

Take a look at any label. It's not complicated once you know what you're looking for. The Daily Value is what the average adult needs each day, in terms of specific nutrients, for a 2,000 calorie-a-day diet. Under Nutrition Facts you'll see serving size, servings per container, calories *per serving*, and fat calories *per serving*. It also breaks down the exact amount of total fat and saturated fat grams, cholesterol, sodium, carbohydrates, and dietary fiber, and protein, as well as vitamins and minerals. Therefore, if there are five servings in the container, and you eat the whole container, you must multiply the calories per serving times five for the correct total. A bag of potato chips, for example, usually has about five servings in it. On the label it says 140 calories—not too bad. But the calories are listed *per serving*, and before you know it the whole bag is gone. Whoops. You've just gobbled 700 fat, cholesterol, and calorie-laden calories. But because we tend to have selective memories and read only what we want to read, we'll focus on the 140 and ignore that it's for one serving. This is a serious problem, because we're so often stymied by our inability to lose weight, when in truth we're eating far more than we think we are.

Food labels by law must list ingredients in descending order of weight. If flour is the first ingredient listed, then there's more flour than anything else in the product. (If sugar is listed first . . . well, you don't need me to tell you what's in the bag!) Likewise, the ingredient listed last is there in the smallest proportion.

Go into the kitchen and get out a one-cup measure and a box of cereal. Now measure three-quarters of a cup of cereal and dump it into a bowl. Most of us eat at least three to four times as much, but because our version of serving size and the manufacturer's version of serving size are widely different, we think we're only eating a quarter of the calories. Not only are the portion sizes listed on packages far below what a normal hungry person wants in her bowl in the morning, they're often misleading. Let's say you buy a cereal that says "No refined sugar—fruit juice sweetened only." Well, what do you think fruit juice is? *Sugar.* Your body can't tell the difference between the fruit juice sugar and plain old white sugar. Eat too much of it and it'll make your hips look like a sugar bowl.

Try measuring your food at home, and you'll soon find the portions getting a lot smaller—and hopefully tempting you to fill up on vegetables and grains. Of course, no one is going to be going out to restaurants with a set of measuring cups in her purse. A handy guideline for food quantities is that a "serving" is about the same size as your fist, or a deck of cards. Make it a guessing game, and have your family join in. After you become used to portion sizing, it'll be much easier to guess when you go out.

Remember, just because the food's on your plate doesn't mean you have to eat it.

BUYER BEWARE

While the government is trying to help us see what exactly we're eating with these labels, cunning food manufacturers have another agenda. And that's to get you to buy their products. One way is to say "Lite," which means nothing. "Light" *does* mean something; to be called *light*, a product must have cut one-third to one-half of the calories of the original food. "All-natural" is another meaningless term. (Butter is 100 percent "all-natural" fat! Poison ivy is an "all-natural" plant!) Another scam is to trumpet "nondairy." Well, the nondairy creamer you put into your coffee every morning instead of whole milk might not have any dairy fat, but it's certainly nothing but plain old saturated fat and chemicals. And yet another trick is really deceptive. This is claiming to be "95 percent fat free," for example. (You'll see this most often on cold cuts.) All this means is that, by *weight*, the food is no more than 5 percent fat. But let's not forget that up to half of this weight is water, which doesn't have any calories. Some of these meats can have, in reality, nearly half of their calories as fat.

All this conniving can really be misleading and very damaging to our eating program. Be sure to read the specifics on the label to see the exact amount of fat grams per serving, so you don't get fooled.

Fat-Free Doesn't Mean Calorie-Free

What Do We Need Fat for, Anyway?

After all that discussion about avoiding fat, it seems contradictory to say it was not so very many generations ago that most people faced famine at some point in their lives, and so we're genetically programmed automatically to store fat as efficiently as possible in times of plenty, so it can be readily available in times of want. Unfortunately, we're still storing fat even though the closest thing to famine we'll probably face in our lifetimes is when there's a blizzard outside and we can't drive to the store!

Our bodies need fat for good health: for energy, to maintain the structure of our cells for temperature control, and for vitamin storage. As women we especially need it when we're pregnant and breast-feeding our babies, which is why we have an extra layer of fat (usually stored on our hips and behind—just where we don't want it!) that men don't. Since one gram of fat is loaded with nine calories, it's a very economical way to store energy. Fat cells also engorge themselves with lovely little bits of fat to keep it readily available. This fat forms cushions around our organs, to protect them from injury. It also keeps us nice and insulated at the right temperature. Vitamins like A, D, E, and K that are fat soluble are transported by and stored in fat for future use as well.

There are three types of fat: saturated, monosaturated, and polyunsaturated. Saturated fats (found in animal products like butter, cheese, meat, as well as palm oils) are solid at room temperature. Monounsaturated fats (olive, canola, peanut oils) and polyunsaturated fats (corn, cottonseed, soybean, safflower, vegetable oils) are liquid at room temperature.

It bears repeating: All fats have nine calories per gram.

Since you must eat a tiny bit of fat every day for optimal health, the best type of fat to eat is *unsaturated*. Your body can't make this. It can, however, make saturated fats—and it does this *every time* you eat too much sugar or protein. The excess is simply converted to and stored as saturated fat.

Unsaturated fats can help lower cholesterol, but only if they're within the 20 percent of your total calorie range. Eat too much, and up goes the cholesterol. What's worse, the process that makes margarine and shortening solid (hydrogenation) has been shown to contribute to heart disease. If your label says "partially hydrogenated vegetable oils," that fat is just as artery-clogging as saturated fats.

Excess fat comes from excess eating. Fat clogging your cells and your arteries gets there when you put it there. Just so you can see how much fat you might be eating, I'm giving a short list here of the calorie, fat grams, and the percentage of calories from fat in some popular items from McDonald's:

Fast Food	Calories	Fat grams	% Calories from Fat
Egg McMuffin	290	11.2	35
Biscuit with bacon, egg, cheese	440	26.4	54
Big Mac	560	32.4	51
Quarter Pounder with cheese	520	29.2	50
Filet-O-Fish	440	26.1	53
French fries (large)	400	21.6	49
Chicken McNuggets	290	16.3	50
Hot mustard sauce	70	3.6	46
Chocolate shake	390	10.6	24

Of course, there are healthier choices, like a plain hamburger (260 calories, with 9.8 fat grams) or the McLean Deluxe (320 calories, with 10 fat grams), but this amount of fat is still pretty frightening. Burger

King (a Chicken Sandwich has a whopping 688 calories and 40 grams of fat) and Wendy's (Triple Hamburger with cheese is 1,040 calories, with 68 fat grams!), and all the others are no better.

Let me also warn you about salad dressings, which are probably the single most fattening food item you eat. One ounce equals two tablespoons, and most packets contain two ounces, or four tablespoons—and are nothing but fat, sodium, sugar, and water. One ounce of Bleu Cheese, Italian, Ranch, French, and Thousand Island dressings has about 130 to 140 calories, and 80 to 95 percent fat. Even reduced-fat dressings can be surprisingly high in calories, because we use so much of them. (Watch a salad-dressing commercial and you'll see them pour about half a bottle on a salad bowl!) Learn to eat salads with lemon juice, vinegar, and a hint of oil, or with very low-fat dressings.

Whatever you do, stay away from movie popcorn. A medium bucket of popcorn popped in oil has an average of 700 to 970 calories, and up to forty grams of saturated fat (from the tasty coconut oil)—and that's *without any topping*. Bring in your own air-popped bag if you need to munch, or suck on a hard candy instead.

Keep in mind that fats have the most staying power in your body; in other words, they're what fill you up and keep you satiated. (Fats also add a lot of flavor.) That's why I think it's so easy to overeat on fat-free foods like cookies and cakes. The fat has been replaced with sugar, but the food item itself doesn't seem filling, so it's easy to overindulge. And each fat-free cookie still has about 45 to 60 calories, which is nearly as many as the original version. If you're going to eat something you really want, go ahead and eat the real thing—in very small quantities. Then you'll be less tempted to binge (see the section "Cravings" later in this chapter).

All About Cholesterol

As with fat, your body needs and makes cholesterol. Cholesterol is a fatty substance found in certain foods and made by your liver. It's a vital component of your cell membranes and your skin—our female hormones, estrogen and progestrone, are made from it—and circulates in your bloodstream. There are two kinds of cholesterol: the "good" kind you want to have and the "bad" kind you don't. Good cholesterol is referred to as HDL, or high density lipoprotein; it can help clear out the LDL cholesterol. The bad kind is LDL, or low-density lipoprotein. Too much LDL builds up as plaque in your bloodstream, sticks to, and then clogs arteries. As you know, this causes heart attacks and strokes.

The problem is our fat-overloaded diet. We consume far too much HDL and LDL cholesterol in our food. This is absorbed directly from our intestines, right into the bloodstream where we don't want it to go.

The American Heart Association measures cholesterol levels like this:

Below 200	Desirable
200–239	Borderline high
240–above	High

But let's not forget that the ratio of good HDL and bad LDL cholesterol is equally important. You don't want your ratio to be higher than 4.0. If your total cholesterol is 220, you'd want your HDL to be at least 55, so your LDL is no more than 165. You never want your HDL level to go below 35, or your LDL to be above 165, no matter what your total cholesterol figure. If it's above 35, you can breathe a sigh of relief.

Reducing Your Cholesterol Intake

- See your doctor. You'll need to be monitored for several months, because sometimes even fit people who eat healthily have high cholesterol levels—usually for genetic reasons.

  There are several, very effective cholesterol-reducing drugs your doctor can prescribe. But no drug can help you if you still eat too much cholesterol.

- Stop eating foods that contain cholesterol. You don't want to eat more than three hundred milligrams each day. Read your labels carefully, and you'll get an idea of how much cholesterol you're consuming. Foods that are high in cholesterol are: egg yolks; any animal products; organ meats like liver, sweetbreads, and kidneys; full-fat dairy products like cheese, butter, and milk. You'll also want to avoid fatty foods like anything fried, avocado, coconut, and baked goods. And although shrimp and shellfish are low in calories, they're also, unfortunately, high in cholesterol. When you do use oil (sparingly!), vegetable oils like olive, corn, and canola are preferable to butter, lard, and palm or coconut oils.

- Start eating the foods that help lower cholesterol. Anything high in fiber, like oat bran, can help reduce cholesterol by preventing your body from absorbing so much of it.

- Eat garlic. Many recent studies have shown that as little as two cloves a day can reduce blood cholesterol; it also prevents LDL cholesterol from being able to build up into plaque. (Garlic is a great food: some claim it helps fight cancer; it helps kill bacteria and viruses; thins your blood to prevent clotting; boosts your immune system; and is a decongestant. It spices up food and tastes scrumptious. Raw or cooked garlic is the most beneficial, but if you don't like the taste or are worried about garlic breath or odor, supplements made by Kwai and Kyolic have been proven to have at least some of fresh garlic's wonderful benefits.)

- Warning: Don't be misled by labels that say cholesterol free. All this means is that it has fewer than two milligrams of cholesterol. It doesn't mean the food is good for you, and it certainly doesn't mean there's no fat—especially saturated fat, which is stored in your body and clogs your arteries . . . amazing, isn't it.

- Start exercising. This'll not only help lower cholesterol but reduce other risk factors (like high blood pressure) for heart disease.

Increasing Your Iron and Calcium Intake

Iron

Chances are we get all the vitamins and minerals we need—except one. The most common nutritional deficiency in America is iron, and nearly 40 percent of all women between the ages of twenty and fifty don't have enough of it. That means our muscles don't get adequate amounts of oxygen, and our immune system is weakened. It makes us more prone to colds and infections. We feel tired and blah.

Women lose iron because we have monthly periods. We also don't eat enough of the foods that are chock-full of it. It's also very hard to take the right amount in pill form, because taking too much can actually cause deficiencies in the other minerals we need, like copper and zinc, as well as promote heart disease. Iron and calcium supplements also interfere with each other, so don't ever take these pills at the same time of day! Vitamin C, on the other hand, *enhances* the absorption of iron. The best thing you can do is see your doctor or nutritionist for advice and get a plain, old-fashioned iron skillet or wok to cook in. A study at Texas Tech University showed that Chinese food cooked in a steel wok can contain eight times more iron than when it's cooked in glassware.

Foods especially high in iron include: raw oysters, lentils, tofu, dried beans, and red meat.

Calcium

As women we are particularly susceptible to osteoporosis, especially when we don't have enough estrogen in our bodies or calcium in our diets. Constant low-calorie dieting means we eat fewer of the calcium-rich foods we need. Caffeine, smoking, and alcohol intake all limit calcium absorption. As I've said, diet sodas and protein contain phosphoric acid, which upsets the necessary ratio of phosphorus to calcium in our bodies and helps contribute to bone loss. Although lots of fiber is also needed by our bodies, excessive amounts can also interfere with calcium absorption, especially if the two are eaten in one meal (lots of cheese and pinto beans, for example). This doesn't mean you should eat less fiber, of course, but rather that you should increase your natural calcium intake.

Just as the best way to strengthen bones is by exercising, the best way to put calcium in your body is to eat it in *food*, not just take it in supplements. The RDA for calcium is 800 milligrams; postmenopausal women who aren't taking estrogen supplements need at least 1,500 milligrams. Try to increase your magnesium intake at the same time, because magnesium allows the calcium actually to get into bone tissue. Aim for 1 milligram of magnesium for 2 of calcium. Luckily that's not hard to do, because most foods that contain calcium also contain magnesium.

Calcium is not difficult to add to your diet. Nonfat milk powder sprinkled into casseroles, soups, meat loaf, homemade breads, and baked goods adds flavor and richness with no fat. Nonfat yogurt is a great replacement for sour cream; tofu burgers are a smart substitute for hamburgers. Any dark green leafy vegetable like kale, watercress, spinach, parsley, or broccoli adds fiber and calcium with almost no calories to your meal. Calcium is also found in salmon, seafood, canned sardines, soybean products such as tofu, sesame seeds, and seaweed (such as that available in a Japanese restaurant or health-food store) as well as calcium-fortified orange juice.

Liquidity: Water, Caffeine, Alcohol

Water

The most overlooked power food is not a food at all—it's water. Eighty percent of our body is water. We can live much longer without food than without water. When we're properly hydrated, our blood flows efficiently, our muscles contract efficiently, and our body temperature is regulated (through sweating) efficiently.

Water fills you up. Water actually helps you *lose* weight because it helps stimulate the excretion of excess sodium and fluids. But most of us think about water incorrectly. Those of us who tend to put on water weight and are easily bloated mistakenly think that if we drink less water, we'll be okay. The opposite is true. The more you drink, the better your hydration, and the better your body functions.

Tap water costs nothing (or pennies). But we often don't drink enough. That means *at least* eight eight-ounce glasses a day. Not sodas, not coffee, not iced tea, not sports drinks, but plain old water. If you're working out more or live in a hot climate, sixty-four ounces might not be enough. Drink all day, before, during, and after exercise. Nothing else can quench your thirst and hydrate your body so effectively.

If you're trying to wean yourself off diet sodas—which I strongly suggest doing not just because they're a waste of money and unsatisfying in terms of taste, but because, as I've said, the phosphorus in them can interfere with the absorption of the calcium you need so badly every day—try drinking plain sparkling water with a splash of cranberry or orange juice. Squeeze in a bit of lemon or lime. Or just add lemon or lime to a cool glass of plain water. Try brewing a huge pot of peppermint tea, which is great for your digestion; drink a cup of it hot, and then chill the rest. You'll have calorie-free, sugar-free, caffeine-free tea whenever you want. There are so many delectable flavors of tea available now that it's quite a struggle not to pique your taste buds when you're in the mood for something hot or cold. You'll soon find that once you've stopped drinking diet or regular sodas, it's almost impossible to go back to them—and you'll be glad!

Caffeine

Most of us can't get through the day without caffeine, which makes it just about the most widely used stimulant in the world. Caffeine keeps you up, alert, and going. It's also addictive, which means withdrawal from it is usually unpleasant—with headaches, fatigue, drowsiness, and depression as possible symptoms. Caffeine increases heart rate, works as an antidepressant, and in large doses makes you more nervous, and unable to sleep. Too much of it also reduces bone mass, which increases the risk of osteoporosis as well as hip and other fractures. The American Cancer Society has reported that there is no convincing evidence connecting caffeine to any type of cancer. Nor has it been proven actually to cause heart disease and high blood pressure. Still, studies continue to examine the pros and cons of caffeine, so I think it's better to drink less rather than more.

You'll find caffeine in coffee, tea, chocolate, and all diet sodas. There are no official recognized limits; some people need only a cup to get out of bed in the morning; others seem to be able to down a pot with no problems. The average amount drunk per day is about 200 milligrams, which is about ten ounces of strong coffee, or several cups of tea. (Just so you know, the "average" coffee cup measurement is only five ounces; most of us think of a cup as having eight ounces!) How caffeine affects you depends on how strong you make your coffee and what kind of bean you prefer, how much you actually drink, how used to it you are, your size and metabolism.

If you're trying to cut back on coffee, go slowly. Gradually reduce the amount you drink, and you'll soon find that a cup in the morning and perhaps one in the afternoon are all you need. I also recommend switching to tea, which has one-third the caffeine of coffee; coffee addicts often need the "idea" of something hot rather than the coffee itself.

Tea, especially green teas, are full of antioxidants, which can cut your risk for cancer and heart disease.

There are also dozens of decaffeinated coffees and teas that are satisfying and delicious. Herbal teas rarely contain caffeine and often have many health benefits as well. Some of the flavors are so delicous that they actually satisfy food cravings.

Alcohol

Alcohol is the most commonly abused drug in America. And it's perfectly legal, even though it contributes to hundreds of thousands of accidents and diseases ever year.

Alcoholism, the progressive and chronic (either psychological or physiological) dependence on alcohol, is a serious and devastating disease. Every time you drink, you're putting a poisonous substance in your body that damages every cell and impairs your immune system. Because alcohol breaks down in your liver, its toxic effects are felt there first, leading to hepatitis, cirrhosis, and cancer. Alcohol also hampers your digestive process, so that many of the nutrients and vitamins you eat are excreted (in urine) before your body can use them. It is also dehydrating and loaded with empty calories. One drink is either twelve ounces of regular beer; five ounces of wine; or one and a half ounces of distilled spirits.

There are many reasons people drink, and how much they can drink without becoming intoxicated varies. All I can say about this is that alcohol may loosen inhibitions, but there are very many drawbacks to more than moderate drinking for women—one drink per day a week. Although there have been studies claiming that a glass of red wine each day can lower your risk of heart disease, alcohol has clearly been shown to increase your risk for other diseases, even breast cancer. Pregnant women, of course, should never drink, as it can cause birth defects. Many drugs also have adverse effects when combined with alcohol. And it can make you more vulnerable to depression.

If you listen to your body, you know it doesn't want to be poisoned with alcohol.

Fiber and Bulk Won't Bulk You Up

Dietary fiber is found only in plant foods, is called either soluble (dissolves in water) or insoluble (does not dissolve in water), and can't be digested by our bodies. What happens is that fiber passes through your digestive system quickly, creates bulk, and draws water into your large intestine, taking lots of the gunk out of your intestines and then out of your body. In other words, eat lots of fiber and constipation will be nothing more than a bad memory. But don't go crazy and suddenly start overloading on fiber and bran—your gut won't be able to handle it, and the result will be lots of gas, cramping, and bloating. Gradually add fiber to your diet, and your body will adjust accordingly. Be sure to drink more water too.

"A diet that's high in grains, vegetables, and fruits—which is also a diet that's high in fiber—is clearly protective against colon cancer and possible cardiovascular diseases," explains Bruce Trock, Ph.D., of the Fox Chase Cancer Center in Philadelphia. Soluble fibers help reduce cholesterol levels in your blood and may also reduce your need for so much insulin by helping regulate blood sugar.

The average American eats only eleven grams of fiber each day, but the National Cancer Institute advises that at least twenty to thirty-five grams are necessary for optimal health. The best sources are: whole foods like whole grains (especially oat bran and rice bran), whole-wheat pastas, bran cereals, legumes (beans, lentils, split peas), rice, and vegetables and fruits with the skin on. (What *doesn't* have fiber: meat, fish, poultry, eggs, dairy products, fats, and sugar. It's better to get the fiber you need from a variety of grains, fruits, and vegetables than from supplements. A moderate intake of fiber (twenty to thirty-five grams) will not interfere with your worries about calcium absorption. It's still not known how your body uses all the nutrients in food itself, so that some of the benefit from a high-fiber diet may be from the food and not just the fiber in it.

Salt and Sugar

Salt

We use salt with abandon, sprinkling it on food before we've even tasted it. It's snuck liberally into nearly every canned, packaged, and fast-food item we can buy. One teaspoon of plain old table salt has 2,300 milligrams of sodium, yet we're only supposed to eat between 1,100–3,300 milligrams of sodium each day. Most of us eat way too much sodium as it is—an average of 3000 to 7,000 milligrams—so we must start to cut back. Hypertension is just too risky and is much less common in populations where little sodium is consumed.

Even physically active people rarely need to think about taking salt tablets or drinking sports drinks. In fact, salt tablets can be dangerous, because the excess sodium draws water out of your cells, so you get dehydrated. They can also irritate your stomach. Unless you are running a marathon on a very hot day, stick to plain old water before, during, and after your workout, and you'll be fine.

Don't pour on salt before you even taste your food. Learn to flavor your food with herbs and spices. Salt substitutes are a fine alternative. And if you're eating whole foods that you cook yourself, you'll automatically be cutting down on sodium.

Foods that are high in sodium are: processed meats; cheese; most frozen dinners and entrees; most canned soup and vegetables; salad dressings; condiments like soy sauce, ketchup, and mustard; pickles and olives; and salted snacks like potato chips, crackers, pretzels, and nuts. Many companies now make salt-free food, so always check the labels.

Sugar

As you know by now, fat free is not calorie free, and the ingredient that replaces fat in all those supposedly "healthy" desserts is sugar. Cups and cups of it. According to the American Dietetic Association, the average person eats five pounds of sugar every two weeks! Imagine how your body would look if you replaced those five pounds of empty calories with something nutritious!

As with protein and fat, if your body cannot use the sugar it ingests, it is automatically stored as fat. So fat free is a double whammy. Fatty foods tend to fill us up; sugary ones tend to make us crave more sweetened and nutritionally empty calories that cause serious tooth decay and the piling on of fat. Excessive sugar intake is also a factor in many diseases, because this sweet substance activates our pancreas to produce the insulin we need to metabolize simple carbohydrates. The more sugar you eat, the more insulin you produce, and the more you overstimulate your pancreas, which is one of the most important disease-fighting organs in your body. Too many sweets also deplete your nutrient reserves, especially B-vitamins and minerals. A twelve-ounce can of soda has between 130 to 170 calories of absolutely nothing but sugar.

We also depend too much on sugar (as well as caffeine and alcohol) to give us a lift, an instant burst of energy. It may work for a half hour or so, but soon we're more sluggish than ever . . . so we reach for another candy bar and cup of coffee or cola to perk us up.

Eating too many simple carbohydrates can also lead to hypoglycemia, which happens when your body can't metabolize sugar properly so you don't have enough in your blood, leading to fatigue, dizziness, headaches, and lots of stress on your body. Hyperglycemia is when you have too *much* sugar in your blood. Quack nutritionists tend to overdiagnose both hypo- and hyperglycemia, blaming all your aches and tiredness on low or high blood sugar. If you think you have a problem, you must see an M.D. and have blood tests for an accurate analysis.

What about artificial sweetners? The jury is out on their effect on your health. Some studies claim that overuse of these fake sugars means you actually start craving real sugars, and your sweet tooth'll win every time. Most people use them so they can justify overeating something else. (A typical example is ordering an extra-large *café latté* and using Sweet'n Low. Well, what about all those calories from the whole milk in your coffee?) We also drink buckets of diet sodas—which as you know are nothing but empty calories, often with lots of caffeine and sodium we don't need—that actually increase our appetite.

How much sugar should you eat? No more than 10 percent of your carbohydrate intake for the day should be sugar. That means fifty grams—ten teaspoons, or a little more than three tablespoons—if you're on a 2,000-calorie-a-day diet.

If you have a sweet tooth as I do, try to satisfy it with fresh fruit (not canned fruit packed with sugar). Fruit is easy to digest and full of fiber and vitamins that fill you up; fruit juice, on the other hand, is rarely satisfying and full of sugar. (We rarely recognize how many calories we can drink each day just from a couple of glasses of juice.) The only fruit juice I recommend is calcium-fortified orange; try to drink a small glass if and when you eat a calcium-rich food or take a supplement, as the vitamin C in the juice increases calcium absorption in your body. As you gradually wean yourself from your regular sugar fixes, you'll miss them less and less.

Don't forget, sugar comes in many forms, so read labels; you'll be shocked to see it hidden there as: sucrose, brown sugar, honey, molasses, glucose, dextrose, fructose, maltose, and lactose. Some, like the fructose found in fruit and honey, is almost twice as sweet as table sugar, or sucrose. You need less to sweeten, but the calories are more concentrated. (That's why honey and maple syrup are *not* health foods, no matter what they tell you in the health-food store.) Sugar is hidden in so many foods, even those you'd think wouldn't need it, like breakfast cereals, salad dressings, ketchup, canned baked beans, fruit-on-the-bottom yogurts (Dannon's low-fat apple cinnamon yogurt has forty-five grams of sugar), and frozen dinners. If you're watching your sugar intake, read labels carefully and buy judiciously.

Vitamins and Other Supplements

Vitamins are one of the most misunderstood and controversial aspects of good nutrition. It has been said that the only people who truly benefit from vitamins are the manufacturers making a bundle from consumers who think if one pill is good, then a handful might be better. In addition, there is conflicting information on the value of vitamins. The Nobel laureate Dr. Linus Pauling insisted that megadoses of vitamin C would help cure the common cold; other studies seemed to dispute his findings, then agree, then change their minds again. How can we possibly know what to believe?

Look at the label on the cereal box again. Eating one serving of a vitamin/mineral fortified cereal will usually give you 100 percent of your RDA (Recommended Daily Allowance) for most vitamins. Our bodies must have the RDA of vitamins and minerals in order to function.

These essential nutrients help metabolism, the conversion of fat and carbo-hydrates into energy, and the construction of body tissues. But vitamins and minerals have no calories, so they themselves can't give your body energy without food. Sweating can cause loss of minerals, potassium, sodium, and zinc. Gulping a handful of vitamins will not necessarily give you pep and vigor. One of them—the fat-soluble vitamin A in toxic doses—can even cause severe liver and kidney damage. Toxic amounts of A can cause headaches and bone pain. The use of vitamin A is controversial—some feel older people need more vitamin A. Too much vitamin C causes diarrhea and stomach pains; too much D may cause calcium deposits in bones and muscle tissue, as well as causing kidney damage and bone deformity. And megadoses of water-soluble vitamins like C and B-12 are simply excreted. Don't believe the hyped-up claims you'll read in a lot of magazines or be told by someone standing in line next to you in the health food store without first checking reliable documentation.

Another word thrown around is *antioxidant*. When your body uses oxygen, your cells naturally form byproducts called free radicals. These free radicals can damage your cells, contributing to the aging process and other health problems like cancer. Antioxidants neutralize these pesky free radicals, which is where vitamins come into the picture—because vitamins Beta-carotene, C, E, and the mineral selenium are all antioxidants.

The American Cancer Society does not recommend that you take vitamin supplements, however, because the best source of vitamins and minerals is food. Here are the best sources of antioxidant vitamins:

Vitamin A/Beta-carotene. Low-fat dairy products, spinach, carrots, squash, pumpkin, broccoli, yams, tomatoes, cantaloupe, peaches, mangoes, egg yolks, fortified grains, liver, fortified milk.

Vitamin C. Citrus fruits and juices, strawberries, kiwifruit, papaya, cantaloupe, green peppers, raw cabbage, spinach, broccoli, collard greens, kale.

Vitamin E. Whole grains, vegetable and fish oils, dried apricots, seeds and nuts, fortified cereals, shrimp, fish.

As with fiber, researchers still don't understand exactly how the combination of vitamins and other nutrients in food works in your body, only that food is the best source. Many people take supplements thinking this is a good cover-up for a bad diet—and they're wrong.

Is there any reason to take vitamin/mineral supplements? The debate rages on. Some doctors will say that if you eat a healthy diet you'll be getting all the essential nutrients you need—but how many of us, truthfully, manage to do that? As you'll see, all you need to do is eat the food pyramid's suggested servings of fruits and vegetables each day for sufficient antioxidant vitamin intake, but only 9 percent of Americans do even that. Others say that their intake may be, well, sort of healthy, but the overprocessing of so much of our food means that taking one-a-day supplements can't hurt. Still others swear that megadoses make for optimal health. The only thing everyone agrees on is that taking a very basic (and cheap) one-a-day pill that gives you the RDA of all the essential vitamins and minerals is fine.

Are there any special cases where vitamin supplements might be needed? Yes, if you're on a very restricted diet (which you shouldn't be, unless under doctor's orders). Yes, if you're allergic to or have certain food intolerances—especially for wheat, fruits, and dairy products—so you can't eat all the nutrients you require. Yes, if you're pregnant or lactating, especially folic acid, which has been proven to help prevent some birth defects. Yes, if you're a strict vegetarian, because you may be at risk for low vitamin and zinc levels. Yes, if you take certain medications (again, ask your doctor). Yes, if you smoke (another reason to stop).

Experts also agree that much more research is needed, especially where nutrition is concerned, because the manufacture of supplements is not a regulated industry. Just go to your local health-food store and most of the clerks, who may or may not be very knowledgeable, are freely and cheerfully dispensing advice along with their pill bottles. This can be just as dangerous as self-diagnosis. There are many quacks out there. There are also lots of medical doctors who don't know enough about nutrition—few get adequate training in medical school. If you do decide to go to a nutritionist or any other professional health practitioner for treatment, be an educated consumer. Ask about their training and level of expertise before you go; if they get uppity or sound suspect just hang up the phone and look for someone else. Be very skeptical if they insist that you buy their own supplements. Your local health-food store or national catalogues invariably have 99 percent of these "unique" supplements for much less money. No ethical health practitioner tries to rip off his or her clients under the guise of "healing."

There is no pill that can change your lifestyle or your body. Vitamins can't make up for too much fattening fast food and stress and too little low-fat good food and sleep.

How to Rethink Your Eating Patterns

The Food Pyramid

Most of us were raised with the notion that there are four basic food groups: meat, dairy, grains, and fruits and vegetables. Recently it has been discovered that equal proportions of these four groups aren't adequate for a healthy diet and, in fact, eating from the four food groups may have led to the high level of obesity in America. The four basic food groups have been reworked into the Food Pyramid, which presents new dietary guidelines. The pyramid has grains at the base—what you should eat most of—followed by fruits/vegetables, dairy/meat, and fats, oils, and sweets up at the top—what you should eat least of.

Grains: Cereals, Bread, Pasta, Rice. The base of your pyramid is supported by the foods that fill you up. Grain-based foods are a source of carbohydrates, iron, B vitamins, and a bit of protein. You should eat six or more daily servings.

Fruits and Vegetables. Fruits and veggies are loaded with fiber, vitamins, minerals, and minimal calories. You should eat two to four servings of fruit and three to five servings of vegetables every day.

Dairy and Meat. These are your protein and calcium sources: milk, yogurt, and cheese; and eggs, poultry, fish, meats, as well as nuts and dried beans. You should consume two to three servings daily from dairy and from meat.

Fats, Oils, and Sweets. They may be tasty, but they're not very nutritious. Eat sparingly of cream, butter, other fats, sugars, sodas, candy, baked goods, and salad dressing.

Many people look at the food pyramid's recommended servings and think it appears to recommend an awful lot of food. It isn't. Serving sizes are much smaller than you think; one cup of pasta, for example, is two servings, and you probably eat more than that for dinner.

Here are some serving guidelines:

Grains
1 slice of bread

½ bagel or roll

1 ounce of cereal (usually ¾ cup)

½ cup of cooked cereal, rice, pasta

Fruit
1 medium apple, banana, orange, pear

½ cup of chopped, cooked, or canned fruit

¾ cup of fruit juice

Vegetables
1 cup of raw leafy vegetable

½ cup of other vegetables, cooked or chopped raw

¾ cup of vegetable juice

Dairy
1 cup of milk or yogurt

1½ ounces of natural cheese

2 ounces of processed cheese

Meat and Other Proteins
2–3 ounces of cooked lean meat, poultry, or fish

½ cup of cooked dry beans

1 egg

2 tablespoons of peanut butter

One problem with the food pyramid is that it doesn't get specific enough about the fat content of food. Theoretically speaking, you can actually claim that french fries (they are made from potatotes, after all!) and spinach are in the same group; but that, of course, doesn't mean they're both good for you. It's the same with ice cream and skim milk. If you use the food pyramid as a general guideline, learn how to gauge portion sizes, and determine how much fat you really need, you will find a simple way to eat healthfully.

Let's now get a bit more specific. When I finally got around to changing my diet, I gradually learned how to cut out coffee, red meats, all dairy products, sugars, and processed foods from my diet. It wasn't easy. But I didn't starve myself, or go on binges, or feel deprived. I learned to *listen to my body* and eat when I was really hungry. I learned that to ease my hunger pangs I could load up on whole grains, vegetables, and fish that were tasty and filling. I stopped guzzling coffee and diet sodas all day and drank lots of water instead.

We need to change the proportion of what we consume each day. No more should we think meat and potatoes for dinner, but potatoes and vegetables and a little bit of meat. According to fitness expert Ellen Laura, the proportions we should eat (unless we're insulin resistant; see below) are:

60–65 percent carbohydrates
15–20 percent low-fat protein
15–20 percent fat
At least 8 glasses of water, every day

About Carbohydrates, Protein, and Fat

Carbohydrates

Carbohydrates—full of energy, filling in your belly, low in calories—aren't the problem. What we put on top of them—butter, cheese, cream, cream cheese, you name it!—is the problem.

Carbohydrates are the major source of energy for all bodily and muscular functions. They help digestion and assimilation of other fats and proteins; and fats can't be burned unless carbohydrates are there.

When we eat carbohydrates, our bodies convert them to glucose, which is the fuel used by our brains, nervous systems, and muscles. Some of the glucose is converted to glycogen, which is stored in the liver and muscles. Extra glucose is stored as energy reserves in the form of . . . you guessed it: fat. (So if you eat a fat-free cake that's mostly sugar, guess what it turns into? Glucose . . . glycogen . . . *fat!* No wonder you're not losing any weight!)

There are two forms of carbohydrates: Simple and complex. Complex carbohydrates are starches in their natural form—potatoes, rice, beans, whole-wheat breads, cereals, pasta, fruit—which are loaded with vitamins, minerals, fiber (and a bit of protein). They take work to break down and are absorbed very slowly into your bloodstream. That's why they fill you up and give you energy.

Fitness expert Ellen Laura points out that simple carbohydrates—sugar, alcohol, honey, molasses, corn syrup—are different. They're digested swiftly, giving you a burst of quick energy that soon buzzes off as quickly as it buzzed in, leaving you hungrier than you were before.

Most of our calories—between 60 to 65 percent—should come from complex carbohydrates. To figure this out, take your daily calorie count and multiply by .60 for your carbo calories. Divide that figure by four, since carbohydrates have four calories per gram. For example, let's use 2,000 calories.

Calories: $2{,}000 \times 60 \text{ percent} = 2{,}000 \times .60 = 1{,}200$

Carbohydrates: $1{,}200 \div 4 = 300 \text{ grams}$

*There's been a lot of talk lately about "insulin-resistant" dieters. It's been estimated that about 25 percent of us are genetically insulin-resistant, which means that when we eat carbohydrates, we overproduce glucose, which in turn overproduces insulin . . . which in turn produces weight gain. If you've gone on a strict high-carbohydrate, low-fat diet and either gained weight, felt hungrier than ever, or didn't lose an ounce, see your doctor or nutritionist for another strategy.

Protein

Proteins are made from amino acids, which we need for growth and tissue repair. Americans eat too much protein, at least two to three times what we really need. This means we eat too much fat, since protein and fat are inextricably bound together in the foods we love like steak and cheese. (Did you know that 2 percent milk gets 32 percent of its calories from fat? Worse, there are 3 grams of saturated fat in each eight-ounce glass, the same as three strips of cooked bacon. Another reason why labels are deceptive.) Look at the food pyramid again. Protein only needs to be 15 to 20 percent of our total calories. The labels on your food or food guidebooks will give you the breakdown.

Let's calculate how much protein you need if you're eating 2,000 calories per day:

Calories: 2000 × 15 percent, or 2000 × .15 = 300. Only 300 calories of protein! That's one can of water-packed tuna!)

Protein: 300 calories ÷ 4 grams = 75 grams.

Now is a good time to talk about the pros and cons of dairy products. The good news is that dairy is one of the best sources of protein and calcium, which is easily absorbed and used by your body, as well as other vitamins and minerals. The bad news is that whole milk (and anything made from it, like cheese and ice cream) is high in fat, especially saturated fat. Furthermore, many adults lack the enzyme needed to digest lactose, which is the sugar found in milk. Lactose intolerance causes bloating, discomfort, gas, and diarrhea. Fortunately, there are enzyme tablets you can take if you have an intolerance, and some milk is specially treated to make it digestible. Still, you should try to eat as many nonfat and low-fat dairy products as possible, especially nonfat, non-sweetened yogurt with live cultures in it; the *lactobacillus acidophilus* that makes yogurt tangy is the healthy kind of bacteria your intestines need to digest food properly and prevent yeast infections.

Be sure to stay away from protein supplements. Not only are they a shameful waste of money, but they can be harmful. Excess protein in the body means you produce excess nitrogen, which strains your kidneys and liver, increasing your risk of dehydration. And too much protein means that calcium is not absorbed properly—which means bone loss. Women are already in too much danger of osteoporosis to add another risk factor. Besides, excess calories, no matter where they're from, are stored as fat. Look at the labels of these protein powders, and you'll be astounded at how many calories they contain. The way to build stronger muscles is with Callanetics and aerobic exercise, not hype and powder in a can.

Fat

Unfortunately, fat calories are more readily stored in your body as fat, whereas carbohydrate calories are more readily burned as energy. Fat, as you know, has nine calories in each gram. Carbohydrates (and proteins) have four calories per gram. This means it takes more work to burn fat than to burn carbohydrates. It also means that it's twice as easy to gain weight from fat because it has nearly twice the calories as protein and carbos. So if we eat more calories in the form of carbohydrates, we'll burn more of them.

To eat a truly low-fat diet, only 20 to 30 percent of our calories should be from fat. But we typically obtain 37 percent of our calories from fat.

Goal Weight	Calorie Intake	Fat Grams*
100–110	1,250	20–28
110–120	1,300–1,400	22–30
120–130	1,350–1,450	23–32
130–140	1,450–1,550	24–34
140–150	1,450–1,550	24–34
150–160	1,450–1,550	24–34
160–170	1,450–1,550	24–34
170–180	1,450–1,550	24–34
180–190	1,450–1,550	24–34

*Suggested fat grams are based on 14 to 20% of calories from fat. (Prepared with the assistance of Ellen M. Laura)

It's easier to count fat grams than calories, especially since the labels do it for you. This table will give you an estimate of how many fat grams you should be eating, based on an intake of 15 to 20 percent of your total calories.

Remember that each gram of fat equals nine calories.

Consistency counts! Let's say you eat 30 fat grams each day, Monday through Friday, and then have a weekend binge when the children come over and eat 75 grams on Saturday and 95 grams on Sunday. Your total for the week is 320. Divide by 7, for an average of 46 grams. Hey, that's not so bad, you tell yourself. . . .

Wrong! Your head might be able to do it, but your belly isn't quite up to averaging. All it can do is burn calories as fuel and store the excess as—you guessed it—fat. So starving yourself one day and overeating the next will only add pounds.

Don't forget one crucial thing: Many people decide to start making smarter food choices by switching from french fries to baked potatoes, or from doughnuts to fat-free cookies. But if you load the butter and sour cream on your potato, and you eat a whole box of cookies, don't delude yourself into thinking that you'll lose weight. Too many calories are still too many calories, whether from fat or sugar.

Here are some useful food substitutes:

Healthy Choice	Not So Healthy
• Baby-food prunes replaces	Up to half the fat in baked goods
• Very ripe bananas, grape juice	Up to half the sugar in baked goods
• Liquid egg substitutes	Whole eggs
• 2 egg whites	One whole egg
• Skim or lowfat milk	Whole milk
• Evaporated skim milk	Half-and-half or cream
• Ground turkey	Ground beef or pork
• Salt-free bouillon and herbs	High-fat sauces
• Water chestnuts	Nuts (for crunchiness)
• Apple butter (on toast)	Butter
• Angel food cake	High-fat cake
• Nonstick cooking spray	Fat for sautéeing

Fat-free or lowfat yogurt, sour cream, cottage cheese, and cream cheese can almost always substitute for the full-fat versions as well. Do remember to experiment with all these substitutes before you make a dinner for company, though, especially with baked goods, as altering the proportions of sugar and fat can change the taste and consistency of some of your favorites. Finding the perfect balance is half the fun of cooking!

Eat with a Plan: Sensible and Filling Guidelines
(Prepared with the assistance of Ellen M. Laura)

Whole Foods vs. Partial Foods

Since you'll be shifting your eating habits from too much protein and fat to lots of complex carbohydrates, an easy way to get started is by knowing the difference between whole foods and partial foods.

What's Whole to Eat: Grains, Greens, Fruits, Beans

Whole grains: Brown rice, kasha, oats, rye, millet, bulgar wheat, etc.

Vegetables: Mom always said to eat them, and she was right. Yams or sweet potatoes are great for sweet cravings. White potatoes (baked) fill you right up.

Beans and Legumes: Peas, kidney beans, chickpeas, black beans, lentils, etc.

Fruits: What's better than a sweet, juicy Georgia peach?

What's Partial to Eat: Remember, Less Is More!

Refined grains: White bread, sweet baked goods

Meat: Meat is a whole food for carnivores like lions because they eat everything—even blood and bones. The human carnivore eats meat as a partial food because we can only digest muscle and fat.

Sugar: Is processed from sugarcane. Fruit juice is also a partial food, because it has a higher concentration of sugar and none of the fiber of the whole fruit.

Alcohol: Is distilled from grains.

Think about your diet. Look at your food diary. Do you eat mostly whole or partial foods? Do you eat a sweetened cereal for breakfast; a ham-and-

Swiss sandwich with mayonnaise on white bread, a bag of potato chips, and an apple for lunch; a snack of frozen yogurt and cookies, several cups of coffee, and several cans of soda; and a cheeseburger with fries for dinner? No wonder you're always hungry. There's nothing there to fill you up. That's why it's so much easier to overeat on partial foods than on whole foods. Whole foods are nutritionally more complete and satisfy our bodies more quickly; our brains receive the signal to stop eating because their needs have been met.

How Many Servings to Eat

For a diet of 1,100 to 1,400 calories a day, eat the smaller serving size. For a diet of 1,400 to 2,000 calories a day, eat the larger serving sizes.

Breakfast
1–2 servings Carbohydrates

1 serving Dairy

1–2 servings Fruit

Lunch
1–2 servings Protein

3–4 servings Vegetables

2–3 servings Carbohydrates

1–2 servings Fruit

1 serving Dairy

1–2 servings Fat

Snacks—2 each day
1 serving Fruit

Dinner
1 serving Protein

3–4 servings Vegetables

1–2 servings Carbohydrates

1–2 servings Fruit

1 serving Dairy

1 serving Fat

Sample Menu 1,100–1,400 Calories

Breakfast

½ cup old-fashioned oatmeal or 1 cup All-Bran cereal

½ banana

1 cup nonfat milk

Lunch

3 oz chicken breast, no skin

2 cups carrots, squash, onions, broccoli

1 cup pasta—tossed with vegetables, ½ oz parmesan cheese, 1 tsp olive oil

Snack

1 apple (midday)

1 peach (evening)

Dinner

3 oz grilled swordfish

½ cup roasted white potatoes

3 cups green beans and stewed tomatoes sautéed in 1 tsp. olive oil

1 cup nonfat frozen yogurt with 1 cup fresh strawberries

To give yourself some variation on this meal plan, take a look at this Serving-Substitution Chart. It will give you a good idea of what serving sizes to eat at each meal:

SERVING-SUBSTITUTION CHART
(Foods listed are one serving size)

Protein	Starch	Dairy	Vegetable	Fruit	Fat
chicken, no skin, 3 oz	bread, 1 slice	skim milk, 1 cup	broccoli, ½ cup	apple, 1 small	1 tsp olive/canola oil
beef, lean, 3 oz	bagel, 5"	yogurt, nonfat, 1 cup	cabbage, 1 cup	applesauce, ½ cup	1 tsp margarine
turkey, no skin, 3 oz	cereal (no sugar), 1 cup, cooked	cottage or ricotta, lowfat, ½ cup	carrots, ½ cup	banana, ½	1 tbsp mayonnaise
sole, 3 oz	cereal (no sugar), dry, 1 cup	frozen yogurt, nonfat, ½ cup	cauliflower, 1 cup	blueberries, ½ cup	1 tsp butter
trout, 3 oz	pita bread ½	mozzarella, low-fat, 1 oz	celery, 1 cup	cantaloupe, ¼	1 tbsp sour cream
swordfish, 3 oz	potato, baked, ½	sour cream, lowfat, 1 tbsp	cucumber, 1 small	cherries, ½ cup	avocado, ⅛
bluefish, 3 oz	peas, green, ½ cup	cream cheese, lowfat, 1 tbsp	greens, ½ cup	dates, 2	nuts, ½ oz
tuna, in water, 3 oz	parsnips, ½ cup	parmesan cheese, ½ oz	lettuce, 2 cups	grapefruit, ½	olives, 10
scallops, 3 oz	popcorn, no oil, 3 cups		mushrooms, 1 cup	lemon or lime, 2	1 tbsp cream cheese
shrimp, 3 oz	pasta, ½ cup, cooked		onion, ½ cup	orange, 1	
haddock, 3 oz	millet, ½ cup, cooked		snow peas, 1 cup	orange juice, 4 oz	
halibut, 3 oz	kasha, ½ cup, cooked		spinach, 1 cup	papaya, 1 cup	
lobster, 3 oz	rice, ½ cup, cooked		summer squash, 1 cup	peach, fresh, 1 med.	
flounder, 3 oz	yam, ½ cup, cooked		tomato, 1 whole	pear, fresh, ½	
salmon, 2 oz	corn, ½ cup, kernels		tomatoes, ½ cup, stewed	pineapple, ½ cup	
crabmeat, 3 oz	pretzel, 1 oz, unsalted		zucchini, 1 cup	plum, 1	
ham, lean, 2 oz	2 Fig Newton cookies			raisins, 1 tbsp	
veal, lean, 2 oz				raspberries, ½ cup	
lamb, lean, 2 oz				strawberries, ½ cup	
lentils, ⅔ cup				watermelon, 1 cup	
kidney/red/black beans, ⅔ cup				fruit jelly (no sugar), 1 tbsp	
garbanzos, ½ cup					

(Prepared with the assistance of Ellen M. Laura)

Callan's Commandments

To help make your eating plan easier, remember:

1. Eat when you're hungry; stop eating when you're satisfied.
2. Eat whole foods; avoid partial foods; avoid processed, packaged foods.
3. Fat free is not calorie free.
4. No fried foods.
5. If you eat something high fat/high sugar (a chocolate truffle, french fries), then don't eat that or any other high fat–high sugar food for at least two days afterward. Remember, fat can stimulate your cravings for *more* fat and sweets.
6. Consistency counts.
7. Limit alcohol to two glasses of wine or beer per week.

Listen to Your Body

Trust your body's instincts about food, and listen to it. It may seem silly at first, but ask yourself if you feel like something hot or cold, salty or sweet, bland or spicy, solid or liquid. You might actually not even be hungry. If your body tells you to go for a walk instead of scarfing down a sandwich at your desk, then go for a walk! Or do some Callanetics stretches. Our women's intuition is powerful (sometimes frightening), but it should not be disregarded.

Don't forget to pay attention to foods that make you feel better. Do you find yourself craving a huge juicy slice of watermelon on the first really hot day of summer? Or a hot, steaming baked potato and a bowl of stew when there's a blizzard outside? Your body is trying to tell you something!

Make changes very gradually. A lifetime of unhealthy eating habits can never change overnight, nor should it. Gradual changes, like switching from whole milk to 2 percent to 1 percent to skim milk, are much more palatable, which means you'll end up with positive, lifelong habits instead of deprivation and bingeing.

Always work at your own pace!

Shop with a Plan
(Prepared with the assistance of Ellen M. Laura)

Never go shopping when you're hungry. It's too easy to give in to temptation and find your fingers twitching toward those impulse buys—you know, the candy bars that just happen to be so temptingly arrayed near the checkout stand when you're stuck in line.

Shop only once or twice a week for groceries. Make a list and stick to it. Stock up on staples when they're on sale. Use coupons.

Here are guidelines for what you should be buying and have stocked in your pantry:

Grains

Whole-grain, lowfat cereals (no sugar added, low sodium)

Whole-grain pastas and bread (no sugar added, low sodium)

Brown rice, wild rice, rice pilaf mixes (low sodium)

Kasha, millet, bulgar, tabouli, couscous, oatmeal

Greens

Vegetables, fresh and frozen (no sauces, please). Deeply colored vegetables, like beets, broccoli, peppers, tomatoes, sweet potatoes, and carrots, have the highest concentration of nutrients.

Fruit, fresh and frozen. Again, deeply colored fruits like citrus, melons, peaches and nectarines, plums, mangoes, and papaya are the best.

Beans

Dried peas, beans, lentils.

Canned beans (kidney, pinto, northern, garbanzo, fava, etc.; low sodium, no fat added. This means stay away from canned refried beans!)

Nonfat and Low-Fat Proteins

Nonfat dairy products (milk, yogurt, sour cream, cream cheese), low-fat or nonfat cheese, tofu, canned tuna (water packed, low sodium), lean cuts of meat, chicken, turkey, fish, frozen yogurt (preferably sugar free)

Condiments

Mustard, vinegar, soy sauce (low sodium), mayonnaise (nonfat only!), nonfat salad dressing, tomato sauce (nonfat, sugar free, low sodium), salsa, cooking oil sprays (they really do work), vegetable and chicken stocks, (lowfat, low sodium), canned or frozen soups (if they have no added sugar, no preservatives, no fat, and low sodium), rice cakes and air-popped popcorn, pretzels (no salt)

Callan's Do-I-Really-Want-This-on-My-Hips (What-Not-to-Buy) Shopping List

Mayonnaise

Whole milk

Butter and margarine

Cola drinks, diet or otherwise

Olives

Candy

Salad dressing

Cheese

Nuts and seeds

Avocados

Fried anything

White flour

The skin on the chicken

Alcohol

Once you start eating healthy, you may notice a reduction in your food bill. Red meat costs more than chicken and fish. Bakery cakes cost more than fruit. Sweetened breakfast cereals cost more than whole grains. Mayonnaise costs more than mustard; bottled salad dressings cost more than oil and vinegar. Cooking yourself costs much less than eating out at fast-food restaurants.

Being able to enjoy your food is a priceless pleasure.

Food Choices

This chart is a good guide when you want a snack. Even though there are foods that are better for you than others, quantities and portion control are good guidelines to healthier eating. A slip once in a while is okay, but there are better choices to satisfy your cravings.

Not So Hot	Pretty Okay	Better
Sweet roll or doughnut	Bagel with low-fat cream cheese	Whole-grain toast with fruit marmalade
Sweetened cereal with whole milk	Unsweetened whole-wheat cereal with skim milk	Seven-grain cereal with strawberries and bananas
Potato or corn chips	Salt-free pretzels or air-popped popcorn	Salt-free whole-wheat pretzels or baked corn chips
Chocolate chip cookies	Fat-free oatmeal raisin cookies	Fat-free whole-wheat Fig Newtons
Fast-food hamburger	Peanut butter and jelly sandwich with an apple	Low-fat peanut butter and fruit-spread sandwich on whole-grain bread with an apple and an orange
Cheese and crackers	Fat-free cheese sandwich with lettuce, tomato, and cucumber (and no mayo)	Tofu on whole-grain bread with mushrooms, carrots, and tomato
Fried rice from Chinese takeout	Rice and steamed green beans	Brown rice and kidney beans with steamed broccoli, green beans, and mushrooms
Pizza with extra cheese and sausage		

(Prepared with the assistance of Ellen M. Laura)

You can balance your food choices by making trade-offs. If you've just got to have fried chicken, then go ahead and cook it or order it, but make sure you eat lots of vegetables (with no butter) as well. Or instead of eating three pieces of fried chicken, try only one. That way you'll have satisfied your "fried" craving yet not overeaten. Eat very lean protein the next day.

Or let's say you want something really sweet. A plain cake doughnut from Dunkin' Donuts is 319 calories, with 21.8 grams of fat (62 percent!); their almond croissant has 435 calories, with 30.4 grams of fat (63 percent!). Doesn't a thick slice of raisin toast slathered with homemade preserves sound better?

Cherly Hartsough, R.D., L.D.N., the nutritionist at the PGA Spa in Palm Beach, is the author of *The Anti-Cellulite Diet* and an expert on food issues. She suggests the following healthy food choices to satisfy a particular emotional eating mood:

Sweet

Fresh fruit

Dried fruit

Baked apple

Baked sweet potato

Applesauce with cinnamon

Fruit sorbet

Grapes (frozen, they taste just like sherbet!)

Crunchy

Fresh carrot and celery sticks

Rice cakes with fruit jam or apple butter

Air-popped popcorn

Unsalted whole-grain pretzels

Low-fat crackers

Smooth

Fruit shake or smoothie

Frozen low-fat low-sugar yogurt

Nonfat fruit yogurt with fresh fruit

Crisp

Low-salt crackers like melba toast or matzo

Bagel chips

Oven-baked (no-fat) tortilla chips

Frozen banana
(tastes like ice cream!)

Fruit sorbet

Warm

Clear consommé with vegetables

Oatmeal or hot cereal

Steamed vegetables

Herb tea

Moderation and trade-offs *do* work and *will* keep you going!

Good Snacks to Eat

If you follow Cheryl's suggestions, here are some munchables for snacks that are filling but not fattening:

Air popped popcorn. (Four cups have only 122 calories. But don't add any butter!)

Asparagus spears

Baked apple (Much more filling than a raw one, for some reason!)

Banana

Cantaloupe

Lima beans (They really fill you up.)

Pretzels (No-salt, whole wheat, hard and crunchy and satisfying to eat.)

Strawberries

Try to Make Lunch Your Biggest Meal of the Day

For most people, the most practical way to balance food intake during the day is to eat 25 percent for breakfast, 50 percent for lunch, and 25 percent for dinner. This isn't always so easy, especially if dinnertime is family time and you're famished after a long, hard day at work. Once you've rethought your eating patterns, though, you can still enjoy dinnertime—you simply won't be eating as much. Leftovers from a wonderful dinner make an equally wonderful lunch.

Some tips from *The Most Fattening Thing You Can Do Is Go on a Diet* include: If you are a stress eater, though, lunch can be an ordeal in the office. Avoid eating at your desk; find a quiet place away from the piles of your workload. Or switch desks with a coworker so you can both have a place to eat away from work. This helps break the habit of thinking that work and eating must go together.

Here's what you should keep as a survival kit for your desk, so that you'll always have healthy items handy for food-craving emergencies: fresh fruit, especially a fiber-rich and filling apple or banana; a bag of air-popped popcorn; salt-free pretzels; a raisin bagel; rice cakes; and sugar-free hard candies (I love butterscotch). Individual packets of your favorite fat-free salad dressing are really useful if you often go out to salad bars.

Don't Skip Meals

Some days you'll be running around like crazy and feel hungry all day. Try to fill up on complex carbohydrates. Other days you just won't have any appetite at all. This is perfectly normal. *Listen to your body.* Eat only when your belly is telling you it needs food (not when your head tells you it wants a candy bar). Nothing's wrong with eating breakfast for dinner. In fact, sometimes it can be downright satisfying to have a bowl of oatmeal for lunch. Start your day with a satisfying breakfast. But if you're the kind of person who just can't eat when she gets up, that's fine. Have a piece of fruit or half a bagel or a cup of nonfat yogurt when you're ready for it. (Just don't ever skip putting something in your stomach!)

Nor should you try to satisfy your hunger with only fruits and salads early in the day. This makes it much easier to overeat in the evening. Some people like to snack, because it makes them feel full; others feel bloated if they eat more than three times a day. Do whatever makes you feel best.

Skipping meals leads to bingeing. We're all going to have a binge at some time or another. So don't beat yourself up when it happens. First, address the situation dispassionately. After overeating, I look at myself in the mirror and say, "Well, Callan, you've just consumed more calories than your body could burn." Period. End of discussion. No scolding. No screaming recriminations. Notice that the dreaded words "should not" are nowhere to be found!

If you can find the trigger that set off the binge, you may be able to stave off the next one. Be kind to yourself. When you feel the urge to binge, try to hold off for fifteen minutes. If you're at work, escape to the bathroom, take some very deep cleansing breaths, then stretch your body all over. Splash cold water on your face. Smile. You're fine. And if you're at home, lie down and do some of the Callanetics stretches, very slowly, in triple slow motion. Or take a walk. Have a bath. (It's very hard to eat when you're wet!) Hobbies that involve your hands are also a great way to keep your fingers busy and away from your mouth. (It's even harder to eat when you're knitting!)

Another useful trick is to change the place where you tend to binge. Lots of people eat standing up in the kitchen; others have to be in their favorite chair, watching television. Even at mealtimes you should only be eating sitting down, in your kitchen or dining room. Those are food rooms. Wherever the TV is becomes an automatic binge room.

When you eat, *always eat slowly, in triple slow motion.* "Food is energy," explains Cheryl Hartsough, "so if you eat food at a rapid pace, then you'll put more stress on your body. Stress creates stress. Learn how to pace yourself." Train yourself to inhale deeply before you take each bite. This may sound silly, but the actual smell of food goes right to your brain and helps satisfy your appetite without calories—so you'll want to eat less. (You'll have tricked yourself into thinking that you've already eaten.) Take very small bites, put your fork down between each bite, and be sure to chew everything thoroughly. If you wolf down your food, chances are you won't have any idea of how much you ate or how it tasted or even if it's enough—and so you'll tend to overeat. (This is where your food diary will help.) Food isn't just fuel. Learn to savor it.

Be Realistic About Cooking

If your idea of carbohydrates is white bread, then getting used to eating brown rice and grains can be a bit of a struggle. Start off with something you like—pasta with a tomato and vegetable sauce (and no cheese) instead of pasta with a creamy cheese sauce, for example. Make your favorite chili recipe without the meat. Bake your chicken and potatoes instead of frying them. Replace sour cream with fat-free sour cream.

If you don't have a lot of time to cook—and who does?—then try to set aside one evening a week to cook and freeze several portions. Soup is ideal for this. If you cook once or twice a week, then you can eat left-overs or eat out for the rest of the week. Try roasting or broiling one or two chickens (freezing most of it in three-to-four-ounce portions), making a baked-yam-and-apple casserole, and a large pot of brown rice. Steam a few vegetables or boil water for pasta during the week, and that's it. Or maybe you can whip up a vegetarian lasagna. It's not complicated. Enjoy your time in the kitchen—make cooking as much a meditation as Callanetics.

Making Food Tastier

- The stronger the flavor of your food, the stronger its power to reduce your hunger and satisfy the rumblings in your belly. One of the reasons spicy food is so great to eat is that it's hard to wolf it down. We savor each delicious bite.

- Trim all fat off your meat before you cook it. Take the skin off your chicken and turkey and fish before you cook it. Skim the fat off your gravies and soups. There are many cuts of beef and pork available now that are just as lean as poultry, so you have a wide variety to choose from.

- You don't need to cook in fat to make your food delicious. The vegetable and oil sprays (plus a good nonstick skillet) really work, so you don't need to sauté anything in tablespoons of butter. Stir-fry with a bit of vegetable or chicken stock instead of olive oil. Learn how to roast or grill your food.

Stay Off the Scale

The scale is not your enemy. Your obsession with it is. If you choose to use it, do *not* get on it more than once a week to monitor your progress. Remember, the scale can't differentiate among fat, water, and muscle weight . . . so as your muscle weight increases, your actual body weight might too. What's important is how you feel and look—how your clothes fit—not numbers on a scale.

Cravings

Woman does not live by bread alone.

Another way to give in to temptation is, as Oscar Wilde once said, to yield to it—but in moderation. So go ahead and put a list of your favorite foods on your refrigerator. When you can't hold off any longer, eat something from that list.

If you're desperate for a hunk of chocolate—and who isn't—then eat the most sinfully delicious, ridiculously expensive chocolate truffle you can find. And you know what? Because it is so rich, so perfectly unbelievably luscious, you'll only eat one. It's enough. You're satiated because it *is* so perfectly luscious. This way you have your chocolate fix that day but haven't denied yourself the pleasure.

If you want butter on your bread, then put on the thinnest spread of it. You get the butter taste, are not putting artificial anything in your body, and that tiny bit is enough.

Like Callanetics, a little goes a long way.

Cravings are weird things. When I'm really trying to behave, I test myself with an exercise in discipline. Do I *really, really* want it and must I *really* have it now? I think about it. I do something else. I go for a walk, or do anything active to raise my metabolism. That usually works. If not, I wait another five minutes. If I tell myself I really, *really* don't have to have it *now*, and I'll eat it *in two days*, chances are the craving'll go away. And in two days' time, I won't even remember the craving.

My eating pattern, however, is stable and I rarely binge. If you suffer from cravings for foods that are not so good for you on a regular basis, then try this. Instead of waiting two days for your craving-food, wait five or six. It's hard, but you can do it. Then, eat your food. Be sure to wait another five or six days before eating that food again. Gradually, you'll get used to not eating it and find yourself craving it less and less.

This method works especially well when you're weaning yourself off high-fat foods like whole milk. By the time you've very gradually replaced the whole milk in your coffee or cereal with 2 percent, then 1 percent, then skim milk, you'll find yourself so accustomed to the "less-fat" taste that you'll find yourself (thankfully) unable to stomach the richer version. I couldn't imagine drinking a glass of whole milk. Ditto with ice cream. Progress from ice cream, to low-fat, to nonfat, to frozen yogurt, to sorbet (which has no fat), and you'll soon find that a mere spoonful of the rich stuff is now as satisfying as a soup bowl full of it used to be.

If you're still having a terrible chocolate craving, you can give in to it without making yourself feel so guilty you keep on eating. Here are suggestions for chocolate snacks that are low in fat—but most are still high in sugar—with the calories and fat grams in parentheses:

Nabisco Peppermint Pattie (64/1)

Hershey Kiss (24/1.4)

Tootsie Roll (large/112/2.5)

Chocolate Tootsie pop (110/0.6—and it takes so long to eat!)

Snackwells Chocolate Sandwich (50/0)

Alba Chocolate Dairy shake (60/0)

Weight Watchers Mousse Bar (35/1)

Swiss Miss Fat-Free Hot Chocolate (50/0)

Dannon Lite Chocolate Frozen Yogurt (80/0 per serving—measure carefully!)

Jell-O Fat-Free Sugar-Free Pudding (100/0—a good chocolate snack, especially if made with skim milk, because it's chock-full of calcium, takes awhile to eat, and really fills you up).

You'll soon learn to distinguish your cravings from true hunger.

BEYOND CRAVINGS

Many food cravings could actually be the result of either allergies or candida, which is an overgrowth of yeast in your intestine. Both must be diagnosed by a doctor who is familiar with these problems—and believe me, a lot of them aren't. Candida tends to get overlooked by even gynecologists, and allergies tend to be overdiagnosed. Sadly, as I've already said, there are far too many quack "healers" out there who are happy to inform you that all your health problems can go away with some very expensive supplements only they can provide.

Food allergies are uncommon; food sensitivities, however, are not. Certain foods—most commonly dairy products, wheat, corn, sugar, yeast, chocolate, citrus, caffeine, and eggs—may make you feel bloated, constipated, and blah. An elimination diet is the only way to determine your sensitivities, though, and it's often not that easy to do. (Unless you're a pro at label reading, you'd be surprised how many products contain corn and/or wheat, for instance.) It's best to follow the advice of a licensed nutritionist or allergist.

Candida is another silent yet potent problem, because it's so easy to upset the natural balance of the healthy bacteria in your intestine. In fact, when some of my students, who have tightened and toned their stomachs, complain about their suddenly poochy bellies, I often suspect that candida is the culprit. If you are on the birth-control pill, have recently taken antibiotics, notice any changes in regularity, and/or crave sugar, bread, and other yeasted products, see a doctor or nutritionist for a diagnosis. Candida is fairly easy to cure with nonprescription drugs as well as supplements of the "healthy" *acidophilus* and *bifidus* bacteria your intestines need to work properly. Buy these at a health-food store. The refrigerated powders are by far the most effective. Take one-half teaspoon every morning on an empty stomach, at least ½-hour before eating. These bacteria are perfectly safe to take for an entire lifetime.

How to Eat Healthy When You're Eating Out

Even if a restaurant meal is a very special occasion or celebration, you can still control some of the calories without sacrificing a wonderful meal.

- Eat a low-calorie snack like a piece of fruit or toast before you leave to go to the restaurant. This will take the edge off your appetite and make you less likely to inhale the bread basket as soon as it hits your table!

- Speaking of which, don't butter your bread. I learned my lesson in Paris, where the thought of butter with the bread on the table is positively shocking to the waiters and everyone else eating in a restaurant! It's simply not done. (No wonder Frenchwomen always seem to be so thin! They don't snack, and when they eat foods full of fat like cheese, they know when to stop, because the smallest morsels are satisfying because they're so delicious.)

- Don't drink alcohol on an empty stomach, because it may actually increase your appetite. If you do drink, sip slowly while you're eating your meal.

- Drink lots of water or unsweetened iced tea.

- Avoid anything fried or sautéed. Grilled or broiled is best. Ask if it's possible to grill or broil with only a little bit of oil.

- Stay away from anything cheese smothered. If you're ordering a sandwich, avoid asking for mayonnaise or extra cheese. Ask for lettuce, tomatoes, onions, peppers, and mustard instead.

- Order a baked potato instead of french fries or mashed (which are often whipped with mounds of cream) decline the offer of butter and sour cream. Use salsa instead—or just salt and pepper. Savor the wonderful taste.

- Eat the vegetables that come with your entree first, to fill you up.

- If you like pasta, order a tomato-based sauce instead of a creamy, cheese one.

- Eat seafood, fish, and shellfish rather than meat.

- Ask for no salad dressing, oil and vinegar, or dressing on the side. Ditto for gravies and sauces. This way you can add your own (teeny) bit as you like.

- There's nothing wrong with ordering two appetizers instead of an appetizer and an entree. Or if you're not that hungry, don't order any appetizer—just keep away from all the bread.

- Have a decaffeinated cappucchino for dessert instead of Death by Chocolate. Its hot, creamy richness will fill you right up. Ask if they can make it with skim milk.

- Order one dessert for the table. Sometimes all you want is one little bite to satisfy your sweet craving after a meal.

- Remember: Just because it's on your plate doesn't mean you have to eat it. Ask to have your plate removed as soon as you're full—then you won't be tempted to nibble just because it's there. Doggie bags are a wonderful thing.

CHAPTER 4

STRESS AND HOW TO GET RID OF IT

Living is stress. It's been estimated that American companies will lose upwards of $150 million this year in stress-related health costs and lost productivity. That's an awful lot to pay for all the tension, anxiety, nervousness, and panic that never seem to go away. A recent survey in *American Health* magazine claims that 90 percent of us report feeling highly stressed at least once or twice a week; while 25 percent are seriously stressed every single day. We experience stress in our cars with daily traffic jams and engine trouble. At the bank we're told the computer is down after we've been standing in line—more stress. We come home from a miserable day at work, the kids are screaming—more stress. We can't find our glasses or the remote control for the TV or our bones ache when we get up in the morning and we just feel old and out of it—more stress. Our relationships seem to be falling apart—more stress.

Yet conflict and stress are not always such awful things. In fact, through them we learn how to confront and then solve our problems.

There's an old saying that if you want something done, give it to a busy person (who knows how to budget her time effectively). Once we learn how firmly to face the situations that drive us crazy, then we can take the steps to deal with them. Slowly. *Always work at your own pace.*

Still, it's not always so easy to conquer stress and not let stress conquer you! It's very hard to know what to do because something that might be stressful to you—driving on the freeway, perhaps, or spending a weekend with your in-laws, or flying from one city to another—may not be stressful at all to your nearest and dearest, and it's very hard for them to understand why you're upset about something they don't even think or worry about. Or it may be difficult for you to express your feelings about being overworked and/or underappreciated at work or at home.

"There are two big stress markers for people who come to me," says Shirley Babior, L.C.S.W., who runs the Center for Anxiety and Stress Treatment in San Diego. "The first is work. In addition to all the usual problems, companies all over America are downsizing, so people are worried about losing their jobs and finding another one if they have to; and with fewer employees, you have to do more work and manage other jobs. It's a really new period in the job force, and causing all sorts of stress-related problems. I see a lot of people who take their briefcases with them everywhere; they don't necessarily *open* them, but they feel guilty and pressured if they're not working.

"The other big stress marker is relationships. People get very overburdened and have perfectionist ideas about what they think they should be accomplishing. They want to be the perfect mate and have the perfect family and the perfect job—and they leave so very little time in their lives to just *be*. It's a continual strain that takes its toll, because people feel very guilty if they can't fit all this 'perfectionism' in.

"Furthermore, our society is more rootless, so we have less of a support network from our family or spiritual leaders. People find it hard to connect in meaningful ways. This is a frightening time, and we don't know who to turn to for help."

I know that I can't ever solve any of my problems by worrying about them . . . but it's so hard not to give in to anger and anxiety if we don't know how to counterbalance them with anger- and anxiety-ridding techniques. After years of teaching, I can tell from just looking at many of my students how stiff and rigid and uptight they are; their body language is a dead giveaway. I see them hunched over, or walking very quickly, or breathless, or unable to meet my eyes or to look at themselves in the mirror. And then as the classes progress I watch them begin to un-wind . . . to relax . . . to *listen to their bodies*. This is where Callanetics and some of the other techniques I'll talk about in this chapter can help you relieve much of the stress in your life.

What Is Stress, Anyway?

Stress is the response in our body to either the threat or needs of a new situation. Humans are genetically programmed to defend themselves against these new situations by what's called "fight or flight"—to con-front something head-on (a caveman's tasty meal he knows he can catch) or to flee from it (a caveman is a tasty meal for a lion in the jun-gle!). In scientific lingo this is called "alarm" and "resistance." So when we're stressed, our bodies pump out the hormone called adrenaline to help us make a decision; our heart speeds up; we breathe more quickly to take in more oxygen; our blood sugar goes way up; and we start to sweat. If whatever's causing the stress goes away, our bodies go back to normal, although we may feel temporarily exhausted by the ordeal. If the stress stays, however, total exhaustion is a likely result. We have no more energy left and simply can't cope. Eventually this can cause both emotional and physical problems that damage your health. "The quick-est way to shorten life is to run on adrenaline for decades," says Dr. Reed Moskowitz, medical director of the Stress Disorder Medical Services at New York University Medical Center. "It leads to high blood pressure, and a ten times greater risk of early heart attacks."

We have all heard of Type A people. They don't just get mad, they get apoplectic; they're aggressive, demanding, impatient, competitive, often perfectionists who are very hard on themselves if they ever make the teeniest mistake. They can be hell to work for and live with. Ex-tremely ambitious, they don't seem ever to take a moment to smell the roses and relax. Well, most Type A people are setting themselves up for trouble, for it's been shown that they're definitely more prone to heart diseases and other ailments. (Still, there are exceptions—some Type A people seem positively to thrive on high-pressure situations. And many of these Type A people come to Callanetics classes because they know it calms them down.)

But you don't have to be a Type A person to have a stress-related medical problem. Stress affects our immune systems, which means we're less able to fight off diseases and more susceptible to everything from colds to the flu to accidents. It can cause high blood pressure, ulcers, migraine headaches, back pain, insomnia, and bad eating habits. If you refuse to acknowledge stress, it keeps on growing, like a bad cavity, getting worse and worse and feeding upon itself until you are ready to pop.

Increasing Your Flexibility—Mentally *and* Physically

Unproductive Worrying *Can* Stop

How can we cope with stress? Endless worrying feeds upon itself. Either you get rid of whatever's *causing* the stress, or you change your perception and reaction to the stress.

Let's say you have a frazzling commute to work and a Type A boss. You can't quit your job, because you need the money. Therefore you can't get rid of whatever's causing the stress—but in this case you can learn how to manage it. Just as Callanetics uses tiny movements to strengthen and make your entire body more flexible, so you can do mental exercises to make your mind's response to stress more flexible.

The first thing to do is identify what your stress triggers are and replace them with stress busters. In this way you can break the cycle of tension and worries that seems to eat you alive. The Center for Anxiety and Stress Treatment suggests the following:

When you are under stress, what messages are you sending yourself? Are they alarming or reassuring? You can decrease your stress by learning to talk to yourself in a reassuring way. This is what "stress busting" is all about—getting your thoughts back on a reassuring track.

First, check off answers to these questions:

When you're stressed and anxious, do you have these physical symptoms?

Feelings of warmth	Heart palpitations
Rapid, pounding heartbeat	Tightness in chest
Butterflies in stomach	Hyperventilation (fast breathing)
Weakness all over	Tremors
Dizziness	Dry mouth
Sweaty all over	Confusion
Speeded-up thoughts	Muscle tension/aches
Fatigue	Insomnia

When you're stressed and anxious, do you have these emotional feelings?

Fear	Keyed up/on edge
Panic	Excessive worry
Uneasiness	Feelings of doom/gloom
Trapped/no way out	Isolated/lonely
Loss of control	Embarrassed
Criticized	Rejected
Angry	Depressed

When you're stressed and anxious, do you say these thoughts over and over?

I can't do it.	What if I make a fool of myself?
People are looking.	I could faint.
It's a heart attack.	Get me out of here.
No one will help me.	I can't go alone.
I can't breathe.	I'm going to die.
I'm going crazy.	I'm trapped.

I'm not going out.   What if someone is hurt,
                          sick, fired, etc.?

If you checked three or more from each list, you are most definitely stressed and anxious! Now ask yourself:

- Do I worry and feel tense most of the time?
- Do I let stress and anxiety stop me from enjoying my daily life?
- Do I want to make changes and be happier?

Wanting to make changes is the first step toward feeling better. Next, put a check next to the following true statements:

Perfectionism

Do you feel a constant pressure to achieve?

Do you criticize yourself when you're not perfect?

Do you feel you haven't done enough no matter how hard you try?

Do you give up pleasure in order to be the best at everything you do?

Control

Do you have to be perfectly in control at all times?

Do you worry about how you appear to others when you are nervous?

Do you feel that any lack of control is a sign of weakness or failure?

Are you uncomfortable delegating projects or household tasks to others?

People Pleasing

Does your self-esteem depend on everyone else's opinion of you?

Do you sometimes avoid assignments or tasks because you're afraid of disappointing your boss or your family?

Do you keep negative feelings inside to avoid displeasing others?

Competence

Do you feel you can never do as good a job as other people?

Do you feel your judgment is poor?

Do you feel you lack common sense?

Do you feel like an imposter when told your work is good or your family is wonderful?

If you've answered YES to any of these statements, you'll have identified issues that are your own potential roadblocks to a stress-free life.

What can you do to change? Challenge these beliefs. Experiment. Try acting in a way that is opposite to your usual behavior. For example, if you have trouble delegating at work or at home—thinking that no one can do this job as well as you can, whether writing a report or folding the laundry—then make yourself delegate. Relax. See what happens. Chances are the task will get done successfully and it's one less thing for you to worry about.

Keeping a Stress Diary

The best way to help yourself make these kinds of changes is to keep a Stress Diary for at least a week or two, just as you kept a Food Diary. Take a little notebook with you everywhere, and every time you find yourself in a stressful situation, write it down, no matter where you are and what you're doing. Then rate it from 0 (most relaxed) to 10 (most stressed). In this way you'll be able to see what really bothers you and causes a stress reaction.

After a week or so, you'll be able to identify your stress triggers. You'll also notice that your stress levels from 0 to 10 aren't always the same. The numbers will be higher when you are concentrating on your most alarming thoughts, and they'll be lower when your attention turns away from them. This will show you that one good way to reduce the level of stress in your life is actively to turn away from these negative "stress-building" thoughts and concentrate on positive "stress-busting" ways of thinking.

Add to your Stress Diary by listing as many answers as you like to the following negative situations:

What always makes me mad?

What always makes me frustrated?

What always makes me cry?

What always makes me feel powerless?

When am I the least contented or happy?

You should have a pretty detailed list of what gets you upset and stressed. Now, make yourself feel instantly better by writing a more positive list:

What always makes me joyful?

What always makes me feel capable?

What always makes me laugh?

What always makes me feel powerful and strong?

When am I the most contented or happy?

What I'd like you to do is keep copies of these lists in your desk at work and at home. Whenever you are in one of the stressful situations on your negative list, stop for a minute, take a deep cleansing breath, and then immediately visualize the *opposite* reaction from your positive list. For example, if driving to work in rush-hour traffic always makes you frustrated, focus instead on how happy you were when you finally learned how to drive, and the pleasure you used to take in it. Then put on a tape of soothing music or pick up the novel you've always wanted to read, take another few deep breaths, and relax.

Here, for example, are some of the Center for Stress and Anxiety Treatment's stress reducers for situations at work:

Stress Builder: "I'll never get this project done on time."

Stress Buster: "If I stay focused and take it one step at a time, I'll make steady progress, no matter what anyone says."

Stress Builder:	"My boss didn't say 'good morning.' He's probably displeased with my work. And I'll get a bad evaluation. Or fired."
Stress Buster:	"I'm jumping to conclusions. My boss might have been in a bad mood. So far all my evaluations have been positive, so unless I get some negative feedback, I'll assume my boss is pleased with my work."
Stress Builder:	"I made a really stupid mistake on page fifty-three of my report, and I can't get it out of my mind. The report is ruined. I have disappointed everyone."
Stress Buster:	"No one is perfect. I did my best. I'm overreacting to one mistake when the overall report is fine."

You can just as easily switch all these situations to your home: you don't have dinner prepared on time; your husband is in a terrible mood; you forgot to pick something up when you said you would.... *Relax your entire body.* Life will go on.

Here's a stress buster to do when you feel overwhelmed:

Instant Stress Buster. Lie down on the floor, on a carpet or mat, with your eyes closed. If that's impractical—you're at work, perhaps—sit in a comfortable chair with your eyes closed. Make a fist with both hands and tense all the muscles in your fingers, wrist, and forearm. Stay that way as long as you can, for up to 5 minutes. Breathe naturally. Then release the tension, letting it all fall away from your fingers, wrists, and forearms. Next, tense your shoulders, neck, and face, hold this for up to 5 minutes, then release. Do the same with your behind, legs, and toes.

The important thing is to be aware of how physically uncomfortable it is when you tense up. Fully enjoy the wonderful sense of release when you relax. If you practice this stress buster at least once a day, you'll soon be able to do it quickly and effectively whenever something's really driving you crazy.

You can do this with a frown as well. Notice how awful you feel—and your face looks—when you're grimacing. A smile is easy. Nothing brings people more pleasure than a smile. Notice how people look at you if you walk down the street with a broad smile on your face. I guarantee they'll smile back because they can't help themselves, and this will make your day. Pleasure is infectious!

Of course, like everything, replacing negative thoughts with positive ones is not an instant process. It takes practice and determination, but the results are worth it. It's very hard to stop worrying, especially since it seems so easy always to concentrate on the worst possible scenario. (For example, your son is late . . . and you're sure his car has crashed. The truth is he's late because he couldn't find his car keys.)

What Stress Type Are You?

Everyone deals with stress differently, but most of us are either a mental stress type or a physical stress type.

Mental stress types tend to internalize their worries, finding it difficult to concentrate, make effective decisions, and stave off "what-if" scenarios from running endlessly in their heads. Physical stress types have actual physical symptoms: a racing heartbeat, a nervous stomach, jittery hands, sweating or blushing, a lot of pacing, for example.

"Once you know your coping style, you'll find it easier to relieve stress," explains Tina Van De Graaf, L.M.T., assistant spa director at PGA Spa in Palm Beach, Florida. "Physical types need to concentrate on their breathing; exercise, proper nutrition, and rest; and hands-on treatments like massage. They do very well with stretching and some sort of aerobic exercise that doesn't bore them so they lose interest. They can also practice their breathing and meditation while they're out on a walk, or going for a swim, or doing any exercise.

"Mental types do well talking out their problems. What works best for them is positive thinking; mental processes like meditation and creative visualization; relaxation techniques; and a good support network of people to listen to them. They tend to feel more comfortable doing affirmations or meditation when they're sitting in a calm, quiet place. They also need to concentrate on stopping the endless loop of tape running through their heads, focusing on one issue at a time."

Coping with Stress

We have many more coping mechanisms—built-in stress busters—than we might think we do. I've found this list to be a lifesaver whenever I'm stressed. Go through it and find several stress busters that you'll feel comfortable doing. As with Callanetics, you'll be incorporating these suggestions into your daily routine, and you'll soon find that your natural responses to stress will be lessened. You'll *know* you can cope with whatever life throws at you. Once you feel empowered, you *are* empowered!

1. **Breathe.** Take deep breaths. Count to ten, or even higher. Concentrate on your counting, your breathing will automatically slow down, and you'll feel calmer. When I get panicky I say to myself, "Breathe . . . be calm . . . breathe . . . be calm," until I feel better and my adrenaline rush has gone away. Then I can face the situation with equilibrium.

2. **Laugh.** Nothing diffuses a tense situation more than humor. Keep a silly joke or cartoon book in your desk. When something really bothers you, read a few jokes, and laugh. You'll automatically feel better.

3. **Call a time-out.** In Callanetics you know to *take a breather whenever you need a break*. If you're at work, excuse yourself and go to the women's room or a stairwell or volunteer to get coffee—anything to take you away from the immediate stressful situation, if possible. Breathe deeply. Do a few stretches.

4. **Always try to take a short walk or do some Callanetics stretches whenever possible.** Keeping your body moving will energize your metabolism, automatically calm your breathing—you need it to exercise!—and divert your energy away from obsessive thinking.

5. **Exercise!** Not just the short strolls to take care of immediate worries. A proper exercise session will utilize your energy in a positive way, make you stronger, and give you confidence that you can accomplish anything you set your mind to.

6. **Drink lots of liquids.** It's hard to say something you don't mean when you're drinking. Hot liquids are naturally soothing, unless it's a blast of double espresso! Stay away from stimulants like coffee or sodas or even juice; you don't want sugar when you're stressed.

7. **Write it all down.** That's what I do every day. I get my thoughts off my chest, down my sleeves, and into my diary. In addition to my stress diary,

I've found that writing down what makes me really mad or hurt or anything is a sensational diffuser for feelings. Let it all out on paper. When everything is driving you crazy, go into your room, shut the door, and pour your frustrations into your private book. No one's going to read it except you. You can say exactly what you feel, without the fear of angering anyone or hurting anyone's feelings, however deserved this may be. Believe me, this will not only disperse your anger or unhappiness, it will often stop arguments from happening.

I particularly like to write letters to people who've made me feel bad—and then tear them up. Some people like to burn these letters—it's a very symbolic and soothing act, as if you're burning all the bad energy away. Don't use a typewriter or computer—I think using a pen or pencil, when you can make your letters as big and crazy as you like, works better. It also takes longer, so it's easier to slow down, think, and be calmed.

8. Instead of reaching for a candy bar or pint of ice cream when you're stressed, try a complex carbohydrate instead. These trigger a neurotransmitter in your brain called serotonin, which has a naturally calming effect. Eat some whole-grain toast, or a bowl of oatmeal, or a baked potato, or a small bowl of pasta. You'll feel full, less likely to binge, and a whole lot better.

9. Get it out of your system. Some people like to have a pillow to punch or scream into. Others just like to scream or yell (in a safe place where no one's going to hear you and think you are in danger). Sometimes a very physical response can help release the stored-up anger; you'll usually feel quite exhausted afterwards. Take care, though, not to overdo it.

10. Retreat to your private place. No matter where you live, try to carve out a corner for yourself, whether it's a rocking chair, or a section of your bedroom, or even the bathroom. Whenever you feel stressed, go to your private place to unwind. Light a scented candle. Meditate. Don't let anyone interfere with the private space you've created for yourself; it belongs only to you.

Always find the time for this daily unwind, to take an instant vacation every single day. Do whatever you want—read, watch TV, cook, knit, listen to music, go for a walk, lie and daydream, write—whatever you want to please you, and only you.

11. Let's not forget music. Music can affect and soothe our moods and health the same way that color and scent do. Not only does it ease away tension but it can instantly lift your spirits. In fact, I recently read about a study that said that students who listened to Mozart had better test scores in school. Let go of all your worries by closing your eyes and listening to calming music, whether it is classical, instrumental, or your favorite singer.

12. Heat, heat, heat. A hot bath with a few drops of lavender oil in the water will instantly relax you. And don't forget hot tea. A cup of steaming chamomile tea is relaxing and will help you sleep.

13. Find a stress sharer. This can be a trusted friend or colleague, a therapist or mental-health counselor, a teacher, a support group, whoever. Knowing you have someone who will understand, be sympathetic, and most important, *listen without judging,* is crucial to the well-being of all of us. We can't solve all our problems on our own.

14. Enjoy your daydreams. Allowing yourself the freedom to let your mind wander is a natural pleasure and a great way to unwind. You might not be able to escape from the stressful situations in your life, but you can always dream about them.

15. Rest your eyes. Some people put cool, wet tea bags on their eyes, as the tannin in the tea is a natural soother for puffiness. Slices of cucumber work well, too. You can also buy gel packs or use a warm or chilled washcloth, depending on the weather. Lie back for a few minutes in a dark place with something soothing on your eyes and you'll automatically feel refreshed.

16. Cry if you feel like it. It's a great way, like pillow punching, to get rid of bottled-up emotions. Watch your favorite sad scene in a film; reread your favorite sad scene in a book. I always go back to my old favorites, and they work like a charm every time!

17. Meditate and read your affirmations (see below). Learning to focus will calm your mind. Prayer is just as effective. Where would we be without it?

18. Learn how to manage your time effectively. You aren't perfect, and you can't be or do everything for everyone who expects something from you. I firmly believe in lists—otherwise I can't remember a thing! If you write down and make To-Do lists, then you have the satisfaction of checking off what you've gotten accomplished. If your list isn't finished by the end of the day, then start a new list for the next day. You'll also become much more realistic about what you can actually get done in a day, and therefore much less harsh on yourself if you find you aren't able to complete everything.

Remember, however, it always takes less time actually to *do* something unpleasant or boring than to worry about it all day long.

19. Learn to say no. As with time management, you aren't Superwoman, and you can't be expected to please everyone all the time. It's amazing how other people will learn to do for themselves if you don't let them take advantage of you. And once you know your limits, you won't find yourself fighting situations you simply can't control.

20. Learn to let go. The words I dislike more than just about any others are "should have" and "could have." There is no place for the "shoulds" in your life. If you wanted it and it didn't happen, then let go and move on. Life is too short to spend obsessing about what didn't happen instead of imagining what might happen if you open your heart and mind to it.

It is possible to live our lives without having our moments of happiness spoiled by those who tell us they "know best"—but that's easier said than done. As I said, what's stressful for you might not even register with someone else. Only you know what's best for you.

21. Volunteer. This is a marvelous way to find new friends and really accomplish something worthwhile in your community. No matter what you think of your abilities, you have skills that are desperately needed somewhere. Nothing is more satisfying than helping others in need, and nothing puts your life and problems in perspective more than opening your eyes to the needs of others.

22. Get a pet. Pets give you unconditional love and devotion. They've been proven to help their owners live longer and to lower blood pressure; and if you have a dog that needs walking, there's a built-in exerciser right there! Taking good care of your pet will give you years of stress-reducing pleasure from a beloved companion.

23. Take a class. Even at the end of a long day, you'll find your mind totally engaged if you enroll in an adult-education course. It can be something you've always wanted to do, like life drawing or photography or ballroom dancing, or something mentally stimulating like learning a foreign language. Studying a topic that involves memorization is a terrific way to improve your memory as well—you'll find yourself much less forgetful. And the benefit of studying for pleasure is that there are no competition, no grades and no tests you need to pass or graduate. The measure of your success will come from within and from testing your own capabilities. We need to keep learning and growing all our lives. There's no better way to keep your mind fit and strong.

24. Treat yourself. You deserve to be pampered. Having a massage or a facial or escaping for a long weekend from all your regular stresses is a guaranteed stress buster.

25. Play. Playing is not just for children. Never feel guilty—or let anyone make you feel guilty—about your need to play and relax. As soon as you find your sense of joy and playfulness, your worries will diminish. The happiest people I know, no matter what their age, are those who embrace life with a sense of fun and adventure.

26. Listen to your body. It's giving you signals all the time. Feed yourself when you're hungry; exercise yourself when you need energy; calm yourself when you need it.

Affirmations

It sounds simple, but you are what you think you are. That's what people mean by the power of positive thinking. If you believe you can succeed, then chances are you will. If you think and tell yourself you're going to fail, then how can you succeed? If you obsess about what you think you've done wrong, then how can you do things right? Our teachers and parents have not always been supportive of us, so our behavioral patterns become deeply entrenched. I have a good friend whose mother always said, "Don't do that, you'll fall"—so she became terrified of heights as a child and grew up assuming she always would be. Well, when she went on a vacation with her family and hiking was available in the nearby mountains, she went off for a walk—and suddenly realized she wasn't scared anymore, that she wasn't going to fall, that people there were willing to help her through it. She sometimes gets queasy coming down the trails, but her fears have lessened so much that she no longer worries about hiking just about anywhere in the world. She doesn't expect to start rock climbing anytime soon, but her spirit and confidence (and her behind) are in much better shape than ever. All because she confronted her fears.

One way I've found to reinforce my positive feelings about myself is with affirmations. The very concept may sound silly at first, but trust me—they really can empower you. It's simply repeating a thought or phrase to reinforce the power of positive thinking. What you do is write down a simple thought or phrase on an index card (or a nice piece of note paper if you like) and place it where you can see it. I have affirmations on my desk, on my refrigerator, in my car, in my purse, in my Filofax, in my suitcases, you name it. Read aloud your affirmation as you're writing it down, and say it aloud each time you read it. You can write as many as you want and change them every day. I like to use favorite lines of poetry as well—they sound so nice! Here are a few examples of affirmations:

> Breathe deeply!
>
> Every day I am getting more powerful.
>
> I am happy to be working at my own pace.
>
> I am happy to be here.
>
> I am calm and relaxed.
>
> I can accomplish whatever I want.
>
> I love _____. _____ loves me.
>
> I am a strong, capable woman.

I'm sure you can think of lots more. Another trick to help rid yourself of negative thoughts is to write down something positive—"I love my hips," for example—when in reality you hate your hips. Another technique is to write down a list of all the negative things you can think of about your hips until you can't possibly think of any more. Then start over till you can't think of anything else negative to say. Next, write down all the positive things you can think of about your hips. It will take some time to do this exercise, but it will help rid you of lots of bad feelings. Simply writing down positive affirmations about what and who you are helps clear the air of all the negative things we tend to tell ourselves all day long. This is why Callanetics works so well—you have an immediate sense of accomplishment about your capabilities, so it's hard to be self-critical.

The Importance of Breathing

Breathing is something we all do but rarely think about. Full, deep breathing brings additional oxygen to all parts of the body, relaxing your muscles so you can function better. Fatigue and irritability go away. Your heart is less stressed and your circulation restored to normal; your blood pressure goes down. Calm, deep breathing makes you feel instantly calmer. In fact, breathing is a perfect relaxation technique because it forces you to concentrate on each and every soothing exhale and inhale.

I strongly suggest you take a class in yoga, or even singing lessons, to improve your breathing technique. Both stress and focus your attention on proper breath control and are wonderfully fun to do. Proper breathing is something you can practice no matter where you are or what you're doing.

How to Relax Yourself by Breathing

1. Sit in a comfortable chair in a quiet place. Close your eyes.
2. Inhale, through your nose, while counting up to 2.
3. Without holding your breath, exhale as slowly as you can. Try to make your exhale last as long as the count up to 6.

In other words, your breathing should be rhythmic, slow, and steady. Keep going for several minutes. Your inhalation is shorter than your exhalation. Don't hold your breath at any time. If you can only exhale for a count up to 2 at first, that's okay. By focusing on counting as you breathe, you will automatically find yourself calmer and less anxious. You can do this when you find yourself in a stressful situation.

If you need instant calming and don't have time to sit in a quiet place, try to focus on a simple 1–2 breathing pattern. Inhale on 1, then exhale on 2. Repeat this at least 10 times, concentrating to keep your inhalation on the 1 and the exhalation on the 2.

To give yourself a break at work or home, set a timer for a minute (or five, if you can spare them—and you should be able to!). Close your eyes and breathe deeply. Immediately visualize yourself doing something marvelously relaxing and pleasurable. Imagine yourself at the beach or your favorite hideaway. Smell the delicious, clean air and hear the roar of the ocean. Your imagination can take you wherever you want to go.

Some people find scent especially evocative of a favorite place and by inhaling a whiff of something that gives them pleasure can immediately relax.

Callanetics as Meditation

People who don't understand the meditation process often ridicule it, yet it is one of the most useful and powerful tools each one of us possesses for inward and outward calming and mental nourishment. It is very simple to do, needs no props or special gear, and costs nothing more than a few minutes of your time. Am I talking about Callanetics or meditation? Both, of course! They're part and parcel of the very same philosophy.

Meditation is a technique that allows the human mind to settle into a state of profound stillness while remaining awake. While meditating, you can experience a simple state of awareness that is very different from our usual waking or dreaming state of consciousness. A tremendous flow of energy becomes available. Meditation helps you relax by allowing you to focus on one thing at a time. Your surroundings will seem to disappear. (In this sense, meditation is a lot like prayer.) Mastering it will increase not only your feelings of self-esteem but also your ability to focus and concentrate on all other tasks you set out to do.

Learning to meditate is like learning how to eat properly. It's also like learning how to do Callanetics. It's something you may have to think about consciously at first, but once you get the hang of it—what I called unconscious competence—it becomes a regular part of your daily routine, and as easy as breathing. All you need is a good teacher—whether from a class or workshop, or even a tape or a book—and a few moments of your time.

I've often said that Callanetics is meditation in motion. Mastering Callanetics gives you the same deep sense of accomplishment; and most important, it teaches you how to *relax your entire body*. One of the reasons my students feel so refreshed after each Callanetics session is because they have used such profound relaxation techniques on their muscles, strengthening them as they go. Relaxing your body allows your muscles to work more deeply. Relaxing your thoughts with a mental meditation has the same effect. The more you relax, the more you are able to relax.

Here are two Callanetics Meditations to help you relax. These take a bit of practice to master but are actually simple to do, and you'll get all the energizing or relaxing benefits from the very beginning. When you first start, you may want to have someone read this to you, or tape-record it yourself so you can play it whenever you can make the time.

1. Awakening the Body

Find a comfortable position, sitting in a comfortable chair or lying down.

Your palms are facing up.

Take a slow, deep breath. Inhale. When you exhale, feel your body completely relax.

Take another deep breath. Exhale. Allow all the stress to leave every cell.

Feel the energy pulsating throughout your body. Feel your heartbeat and the warmth of your blood pulsing through all the cells in your body.

Focus now on that warm energy as it moves down to your feet. Concentrate on pulling the energy away from your extremities toward the center of your body. Feel the tingling sensation as you start to withdraw that energy from your feet, toes, and calves. Following the tingling will be a lovely numbing, relaxing of that part of your body.

Continue to pull all that wonderful warm energy up through your thighs and hips to your stomach.

Feel your fingers tingle as the energy continues to pull away, traveling through your hands, wrists, arms, and chest, moving to the center of your stomach.

Relax your face, especially your jaw.

Feel your scalp tingle, then go numb, as energy continues to move away from your face, jaw, neck, and then down to the center of your body.

Every cell has gone to sleep, except for the warm ball of energy glowing in the center of your stomach.

Concentrate on that energy.

Feel the warmth increase and grow. It's now traveling in a circular motion, becoming stronger, warmer, brighter, until it forms a funnel to leave the center of your body.

Your body is now in a complete state of relaxation. The energy has spread and draped over you completely.

Its caressing powers nurture you. You are flooded with a delicious sense of peace.

Allow the energy to cover and protect you.

And now the energy is starting to move, like a magnet pulling at your body. Feel the energy circle around your body.

The pores of your skin reopen, as if they are releasing all the stress trapped within.

Let your body heal.

Remove all negative thoughts from your mind. Let go of all judgment and ego.

Fear, anger, resentment, envy, self-pity are withdrawn through this giant funnel.

The energy moves more swiftly now, and in its place you'll feel a steady sense of peace and calm. Your emotions are soothed and comforted.

Your body is strong, whole, and vital. You feel a peaceful sense of energy, strength, and awareness. Feel its pulsating power circling from your stomach to your hips and then down to your thighs, calves, and feet.

Your body is awakening to a pristine feeling of new life.

Turn to your side, whether you are sitting or lying down. Allow your heart rate to return to normal. Now, breathe in deeply, then breathe out. Open your eyes.

Feel your new power.

2. Relaxing the Body

Find a comfortable position, lying down, with your palms facing up.

Take a deep breath, then exhale. Pretend you are allowing your body to relax and melt into the floor. Take another deep breath. Exhale. Concentrate on allowing all stress and tension to leave your body completely. You are feeling more relaxed now, and very light.

The tension has gone out of your body as if you were a rag doll.

Focus on the center of your body. Feel a great, radiant, warm stream of light leaving your center and flowing over you. Spreading its warm protective blanket over you, it is nurturing and caressing.

You are lighter and being lifted off the floor.

Your blanket of light lifts you above the ceiling, the trees, into the heavens.

You are flying over earth. A force is drawing you closer to another land. You allow yourself to be lowered down to that special land.

You see yourself stand erect, with confidence, and look upon a magnificent garden.

You walk into the lush green grass, feeling its coolness beneath your feet, and you revel in breathing in the cool crisp air, the fragrant scent of the flowers blooming around you.

Look around and admire this landscape. Everything is intense, yet calm. You feel a true sense of peace here. The sky is blue, the clouds white, the colors gorgeous.

Your eyes settle on a pond in the distance, surrounded by more flowers and rocks warmed by the sun.

There is a waterfall gently cascading into the pond. You step into the sparkling crystal blue water, like a liquid jewel. You feel your skin tingle from head to toe, the pores relaxing and opening to drink in this magical water.

Peace and harmony flood your senses.

In triple slow motion you dive through the water, eager for more of its magic. You slowly swim to the waterfall and let it flow over your body. You feel yourself changing, as if all the cells in your body were coming alive, reshaping and strengthening you. Beauty and youthful vigor are claiming their right to exist in your body.

Next you swim to the edge of the pond, gently climb out, and sit on the warm rocks. The sun dries your skin with the purest energy, locking the healing powers within you.

This is your special place. A precious, private, secret hideaway.

And you have come back to it.

Lie down on the soft grass. A stream of light from the center of your body once again surrounds you. Look at yourself and feel very peaceful, youthful. Everything in this enchanted land is reflected in you.

Close your eyes and allow the light to lift you and bring you safely back to where you are lying. You feel calm and peaceful.

Improving Your Sleep

Most of us are exhausted from perpetual sleep deprivation, and we don't even realize that's the cause of our profound fatigue. Without a good night's sleep we can never feel truly fit, but how many of us have time ever to get the real amount our bodies crave? The average woman needs at least seven to eight hours but usually has less. No wonder we're too tired to think straight. And worrying about how much sleep we're not getting—along with everything else—leads to restlessness, interrupted sleep, and insomnia.

Insomnia is most often caused by stress and worries, depression, an illness, or poor sleep habits; it's a special problem during menopause when hot flashes disrupt your sleep cycle. It can lower your immune system response so you're more prone to illness. Taking sleeping pills is just about the last thing you should do if you can't sleep, as they don't allow you the deepest level of sleep your body needs to recharge itself and can become addictive. Like laxatives, sleeping pills appear to alleviate symptoms temporarily, but they don't address the underlying cause and only make matters worse.

The Sleep-Wake Disorders Center of the New York Hospital-Cornell Medical Center suggests the following Rules of Good Sleep Hygiene for Insomniacs:

1. Sleep on a very regular schedule, *including* weekends. Regular means climbing into bed and turning out the light at the same time (plus or minus fifteen minutes) every night of the week and awakening and arising from bed at the same time (plus or minus fifteen minutes) every morning. This schedule should be adhered to without fail for at least two weeks before even slightly more variability (plus or minus thirty minutes) is permitted.

   This means always go to bed at the same time whether you feel tired or not, and set the alarm for the same time every morning no matter what time you actually fell asleep the night before.

   If it is absolutely necessary to stay up late for one or two nights for business or social reasons, *do not sleep late* the next morning(s). Getting up at the same time every day is crucial to resetting our "internal" clock. Getting up at the same time every day reinforces this internal clock's ability to foster sleep in the same time zone. Varying your getting-up time, especially by sleeping late, clashes with this basic property of your internal clock and makes your sleep much more fragmented. In other words, too much variation in your sleep schedule can produce a kind of jet lag, even though you haven't taken a flight anywhere.

2. Don't spend too much time in bed. One half hour more than your *average* amount of sleep per twenty-four hours is enough. This aspect of your sleep schedule is just as important as the principles of sleep timing

in item #1 above. In general, the more time spent actually asleep while in bed—this is referred to as "sleep efficiency"—the more satisfying, "deep," and restful your sleep experience is. Spending very much more time in bed than can be filled with sleep produces inefficient and therefore less-restful sleep.

To figure out your average sleep time, simply jot down your best estimate of how many hours and minutes you slept the night before, as soon as you get up in the morning. After fourteen nights, add up your numbers and divide by 14. This will be your average daily sleep time.

You can even design your own sleep schedule by adding a half hour to your average sleep time. Decide what time you want to get up every morning, take your average daily sleep time figure, then work back from this wake-up time by that figure plus half an hour to determine your bedtime. So if you want to get up at 7 A.M., and your average sleep time is eight hours, then count back eight hours from 7 A.M. = 11 P.M. Subtract half an hour = 10:30 P.M. That's your new bedtime.

3.   Avoid drinking any beverage with caffeine, which as you know is a stimulant, after noontime. If this doesn't help, try to avoid caffeine altogether.

4.   Try to avoid alcohol as well, which is also a stimulant, within four hours before bedtime, if not altogether.

5.   Exercise, but do your workout in the morning or afternoon. Try to let at least three to four hours elapse between exercise time and bedtime.

6.   Do something relaxing in the hour or so before getting into bed. Avoid arguments, excitement, and bill paying during this time.

7.   A light bedtime snack (without sugar) is okay, but avoid eating a full meal just before bedtime.

8.   Stop trying to *make* sleep happen. You have to *let* it happen.

I also think you should make your bedroom a safe haven that is only used for sleep and other pleasures. Make sure you've left the day's weariness behind. In other words, you don't want a desk near your bed to remind you of all the bills you have to pay. Let go of your work load for the night—worrying about it certainly isn't going to help you sleep.

Aside from a good reading light next to or over your head, having a soft, flattering light in your bedroom will make it feel cozy and warm.

End the day and start your night's sleep with comforting, positive, and optimistic thoughts. Practice your breathing and you'll conk out before you know it. Before going to bed, soak in a luxurious warm bubble bath. Sipping a hot herbal tea can also help you sleep. Chamomile, valerian, hops, and passion flower all have a calming effect.

This may sound silly, but the color of your bedroom and sheets can have an effect on your sleeping! (This has been proven in hospitals and prisons, where calm colors improve everyone's sleep as well as dispositions.) Paint the walls a soft, quiet color, like lovely pale aqua, rose, or spring green.

Taking Time to Pamper Yourself

In this hectic, overstimulating, frenetically paced world, few of us stop to take the time for the regenerating kind of treatments we not only deserve but need, both mentally, spiritually, and physically. I see massage and aromatherapy treatments not as luxury indulgences but as vital, regular, indispensable necessities for rebalancing our energy. Hands-on treatments from skilled practitioners are very effective and relatively inexpensive ways to unwind not only from aches and pains but from all the stresses and emotions we store in our bodies, wittingly or not. These are the best drug-free treatments I know for a whole range of ailments.

Massage

Massage is one of the oldest and most natural of all the medical treatments used to heal and relieve pain. In the early fifth century B.C., Hippocrates, the "father of medicine," wrote: "The physician must be experienced in many things, but assuredly in rubbing . . . for rubbing can bind a joint that is too loose, and loosen a joint that is too rigid."

Americans have been slow to embrace the wonders of massage, in part because of the seamy sex trade that used massage as a euphemism for something else! With thousands of qualified professionals working as massage therapists (*not* to be called masseur or masseuse, mind you), it should be easy to find someone skilled near you. (Ask friends, your doctor, alternative healers, your chiropractor, check listings at your health-food store, try the yellow pages.) They work on a special table that cradles your head comfortably, and you are covered with either sheets or towels the entire time, so there's nothing to worry about if you're apprehensive about a stranger touching you.

If you want soothing muscle work, go for the Swedish technique, which is very hands-on, with long strokes; or the Japanese shiatsu, which works on the same energy meridiens as acupuncture. If you have specific medical problems, a specially trained therapist can help ease the aches with a medical massage; if you have injuries, a sports massage can also greatly alleviate pain in a specific area. Massage lowers your blood pressure and is fabulously relaxing. There's something about the laying-on of healing hands that nourishes not only your body but also your spirit. Studies have proven that massage stimulates your immune system.

Touch is so important and so healing!

HOW TO GIVE YOURSELF A MASSAGE

Nothing's better than a professional massage for easing the kinks and tensions out of your body, but often we either can't afford or don't have the time for one. There's no reason you can't take some time for yourself and help de-stress your body. Self-massages are especially useful in combination with aromatherapy oils, as these have an immediate effect on your state of mind.

A self-massage will take about fifteen to twenty minutes and should be done in a room that is calm, quiet, and dimly lit. Warm up your oil—it should be just slightly warmer than body temperature—by placing a small vial of it in a cup of hot water before you lie down. Before your massage starts, lie calmly on a firm surface and breathe deeply for a few minutes. This is crucial for relaxation. When you're ready to start, pour a few drops of oil in your palms and vigorously rub them together; this energizes your hands and keeps the oil warm enough to apply to your skin (cold hands and oil are not exactly what I'd call relaxing!).

If you don't mind getting oil in your hair (it's actually very conditioning, especially if your scalp is dry), then use about ⅛ cup of oil and massage it in vigorously with your palm. Next, gently knead the back of your neck with your fingers, using a back and forth motion. Move to your throat, using only upward strokes. Follow that with circular strokes with your whole hand on your shoulders and elbows. Stroke each arm, in long movements up and down. Massage your chest and abdomen using your palms moving clockwise. Don't forget your hips and behind, going around in circles. Stroke your legs in long movements as you did your arms. Finish with your feet and hands, which are supersensitive areas loaded with nerve endings.

Relax! Breathe deeply! You deserve this.

Aromatherapy

Our sense of smell is unique. In fact, whenever you smell anything, it goes straight to your brain, which is why aromas can have such a potent effect on us.

Aromatherapy is an ancient art, first invented by the Egyptians, who were great practitioners of all forms of bathing and created many perfumes. Aromatherapy uses essential oils (distilled from flowers, plants, woods, and herbs) to please the spirit and nurture and refresh the body. You can inhale the vapors of these strongly scented oils, apply them to the skin for a massage, or use them in a bath.

Until you have an aromatherapy massage with scented oils that your massage therapist has mixed up for you, depending on your physical and mental condition, it's hard to believe something that smells so nice can have such a powerful effect of soothing, energizing, revitalizing, or relaxing. These oils can help relieve symptoms of colds and other illnesses, ease aches and pains, improve digestion, strengthen the immune system, and much more.

To have scent around you all the time, you can buy special lamps that diffuse scent into a room for long-lasting effects. There is also a metal ring that you can place around a light bulb for holding a few drops of oil. The heat of the bulb slowly diffuses the oil's aroma. There are many books detailing the properties of each oil, so that you can mix up a batch of your own delectable concoction at home. The great fun of experimenting with essential oils is creating your own unique perfumes.

*Never apply undiluted essential oils to your skin. They are extremely potent, so they must be used sparingly. Only a few drops are needed, mixed into a small amount of a neutral base oil like sweet almond or jojoba or any vegetable oil (avoid extra-virgin olive oil, as it tends to have its own scent—and it's also expensive!).

Instant Headache Buster. This works for some, and I hope it will for you also. Mix a drop of rosemary essential oil with a few drops of sweet almond oil. Dip your third finger in this deliciously scented oil and place it right in the middle of your forehead. Without lifting your finger, massage this area, in a circular motion, for seven to ten minutes. Your headache should go away.

A few drops of rosemary oil in a lightbulb diffuser is also a good way to rid yourself of headaches. It will also make your room smell great!

Alternative Therapies

In my opinion, one of the great failings of modern medicine is its inability, despite all the great strides in drug research and disease prevention, to *listen* to the patient, and to recognize the connection between mind and body. Women's intuition is a powerful tool, yet we rarely listen to it. If we, who live in our own bodies and know how they work best, think something is wrong—or just *off*—it probably is. Don't let anyone tell you otherwise. This is where alternative therapies come in. They believe in treating the cause, and not just the symptom; they seek to rebalance the energy of your body, not find a quick fix. A perfect example of the quick-fix mentality is the overprescription of antibiotics.

In a fascinating book I urge you to read, *Outrageous Practices: The Alarming Truth about How Medicine Mistreats Women,* authors Leslie Lawrence and Beth Weinhouse talk about how women with genuine symptoms and medical conditions are misdiagnosed, ignored, or rebuffed as hysterics by the very doctors who are supposedly there to treat them. "Unfortunately," they write, "women's complaints are dismissed by doctors far too often—and much more readily than men's. One study found that primary-care physicians judged 65 percent of women's symptoms, versus 51 percent of men's, to be influenced by emotional factors. Perhaps not surprisingly, women's complaints were more than twice as likely as men's to be identified as psychosomatic [or 'all in the head']. Misdiagnosing a woman is bad enough, but misdiagnosing her as a result of sex bias is unforgivable. At the very least it can delay appropriate care; at worst it can threaten her life."

The biggest difference I've found between alternative, holistic healers and the medical establishment is that holistic practitioners *listen* to you, and I hope you will be able to talk to them about your underlying conditions because you've learned to *listen to your body.* (Of course it can be just as difficult to find a good holistic practitioner as it is to find a medical doctor you trust, especially if you live outside of a big city.) The down side of alternative medicine is that they're rarely covered by your medical insurance, and you must check credentials carefully. Just about anyone can hang out a shingle and call herself a reflexologist or aromatherapist, for example. Ask for recommendations from your friends; call schools near you; ask about licensing and accreditation. Acupuncture, for instance, has been a regulated industry for less than twenty years. But just because your regular doctor might scoff at some of these practices—I doubt that he or she has ever experienced them—is no reason not to seek help if you feel you need it. I know how much some of these therapies have helped me.

Acupuncture

Chinese medicine is based on a concept of what they call "Qi" or "Chi" (pronounced *chee*), which is best described as the energy of your body. According to acupuncture, the pathways where the Qi flows are called meridiens, and placing superfine (disposable) needles along different points in these meridiens will remove energy blockages, lessening pain and helping you to heal naturally. It is a painless process—sometimes you'll feel a slight tingling sensation, but never anything like a shot from a hypodermic!—and is remarkably effective for chronic pain (like lower-back pain, sciatica, arthritis) or acute pain (a migraine or injury). It also works well for anything from cataracts to bronchitis to insomnia, depression, anxiety, and weight control. The effects of multiple sessions are cumulative, so the more you go, the better you'll feel. It can help you stop smoking and even lessen the pain of childbirth and ease you through the symptoms of menopause.

Ayurveda

Ayurveda means "the science of life" in Sanskrit, and it is based on a 6,000-year-old Indian system of rejuvenation, beauty, and health care. At its heart is the concept of three body types, or *doshas*: Vata (from air), Pitta (from fire), and Kapha (from water). Each person is a unique combination of these doshas, and so an ayurvedic treatment would be custom designed to balance your physical and mental tendencies. Breathing, diet, stress management, and meditation are important parts of the ayurvedic philosophy. I've found that ayurveda students often are drawn to and helped by Callanetics.

Herbal

Herbs have been used for centuries—by medicine men, witches, doctors, and, most likely, your parents or grandparents—to treat illness, dye fabrics, even make cosmetics. In fact, many of our most potent drugs are based on the "folklore" knowledge of the medicinal use of plants, flowers, barks, and roots. As with aromatherapy, there are many books available that teach you which herbs have specific therapeutic properties, and it may be worth your time to take a class at a local health-food store or community college to learn about the wonders of herbs. It's even better to see an herbalist if you can. Herbs are available as powder (to be made into pill capsules), tinctures to be added to water, and in their natural state to be brewed into delicious teas. Some herb potions are blended into bath oils that are either calming or energizing, and they work wonderfully well.

Homeopathy

I'll bet you didn't know that 15 percent of the physicians in this country a hundred years ago were homeopaths. Homeopathy was invented by a German physician, Dr. Hahnemann, in the early nineteenth century, became very popular, then seemed to disappear as drugs were invented. Now many people are talking about it again; even Princess Diana in England seeks homeopathic treatment.

The basic principle behind homeopathy is that like cures like, so that an illness can be cured with a medicine that creates symptoms similar to what you're experiencing. Minute dilutions of the substance are used, which seems to be contrary to the principles of Western, scientific medicines. No one has been able to prove how homeopathy works, but many have found it successful for them. You'll have to try it for yourself to see who's right!

Reflexology

Reflexology is an ancient holistic healing technique to relieve pain and stress as well as improve energy and circulation. According to the principles of reflexology, there are very specific ("reflex") areas on your feet that correspond to the organs, glands, and other parts of your body.

When these points are pressed, there is a reflex action on the corresponding area in your body. A skilled reflexologist can tell you pretty much everything you know is achy or wrong with your body by touching your toes and the soles of your feet. If I had the time, I'd have a reflexology treatment every week—that's how much I believe in it.

CALLANETICS EXERCISES

CHAPTER 5

CALLANETICS

About Callanetics

As millions of women have proven, anybody, at any age, and in any shape can do Callanetics.

With one small movement, Callanetics has revolutionized the world of fitness. Callanetics will have a profound change on how you see yourself and your body. Because it affects how you stand, walk, and sit, Callanetics will drastically improve your posture, balance, and alignment. In just a few short sessions you'll be standing stronger, feeling stronger, and acting stronger. Knowing you *can* change the shape of your body has a intense and wonderful effect on your self-esteem.

What Is Callanetics?

Callanetics is a total system of very tiny muscle contractions and complementary stretches. Even though these movements are as small and gentle as a pulse beat, you're working your muscles very deeply. This is why Callanetics works so quickly yet is a completely safe and effective way to tone and strengthen your body. You will be taught how *not* to put any pressure or strain on your lower back, and stretching your spine will improve your posture. Your back muscles will loosen and you'll be standing more erect so you'll seem taller. Your stomach will flatten and your behind will tighten and lift. I have always said that Callanetics defies gravity—and it's a lot better than liposuction!

You need no special equipment or workout shoes (you can't wear them, as they're too heavy) to do Callanetics—only a leotard or comfortable clothing; a mat or towel to cushion your back, knees, or buttocks; and the use of a barre or stable piece of furniture at a comfortable height for you, like the back of a sofa or chair or a strong table. You can even use a file cabinet. Make sure it is sturdy enough to support your weight.

Callanetics Vocabulary

There are phrases you've seen throughout this book that apply to not only the actual Callanetics exercises but also to my life philosophy. These are:

> Listen to your body
>
> Gentle, delicate little motions
>
> Relax your entire body
>
> Triple slow motion
>
> Always work at your own pace
>
> Never compare yourself with anyone else
>
> Never, ever force
>
> Light and flowing as a feather
>
> Your body is like a rag doll
>
> Let yourself melt into the floor

These are key phrases to help you manage your lifestyle as well as perform Callanetics effectively. If you *listen to your own body, relax your entire body*, and work in *triple slow motion, never, ever forcing,* you'll feel *as light as a feather.* As long as you *never compare yourself with anyone else*, you'll *always work at your own pace* and be successful at whatever you choose to do.

Triple Slow Motion

I came up with this phrase because it sounds so evocative. All the movements in Callanetics are no more than one-quarter to one-half inch — take out a ruler to see how tiny a pulse this is! — so small, precise, and always done very, very slowly. You'll never be jerking, bouncing, or straining in any way. When you feel how deeply you can work with such a small, slow movement, then you'll know you're doing Callanetics correctly.

Counting

When I say seventy-five repetitions, for example, this means seventy-five tiny pulses done in triple slow motion. A "rep" is an abbreviation for "repetition." If an exercise says "hold for a count of . . ." you should count one-thousand-and-one, etc. Counting aloud will also help you to breathe effectively.

Breathing and Taking a Breather

Always breathe naturally — and don't forget to breathe! I'm not kidding, because a lot of people tend to hold their breath whenever trying an exercise that is new and different. In Callanetics you'll be focusing on your triple slow motion, so your breathing should come naturally.

"Taking a breather" means you can gently take yourself out of whatever position you're in, exhale and inhale deeply for a few seconds, *relax*, and then resume the correct position. If a Callanetics exercise is too much at first, you can take as many breathers as you like until you finish. *Always work at your own pace.*

And don't forget — *never compare yourself with anyone else.* Some people are naturally more flexible or have stronger muscles. Don't let their progress or body shape frustrate your own efforts!

Curling Up Your Pelvis

The heart of Callanetics is the concept of curling up your pelvis. Your pelvic area affects your balance, alignment, and posture; loosens up your hip joints; and allows all your movements to be more free and fluid. It is the link between your upper and lower body, a gentle rounding up. When you curl it up in triple slow motion, you are literally trying to bring your pubic bone up to your belly button. Imagine there is a string attached to the bottom of your leotard; if you pull on the string, your pelvis will automatically curl up. The more you curl up, the more you stretch your spine as well as tighten your abdominal muscles and buttocks.

To curl up your pelvis, stand with your feet hip width apart, knees slightly bent and relaxed, toes pointing forward. Your arms and body are relaxed. Tighten your behind. In triple slow motion, curl your pelvis up, aiming in toward your navel. Your upper back will round slightly. Feel the release in your lower back.

Release the curl and return to your original position in triple slow motion.

Visualize a wave moving in reverse movement washing under you as you curl up. Your goal is to keep your back completely relaxed while you're curling up as much as possible.

Practice curling up your pelvis whenever you like. It helps prepare your muscles and spine for all the Callanetics exercises.

Never, Ever Force

You should never try to do more than your body tells you to. Never force a stretch. *Always listen to your body.* No pain, no gain is a fallacy! Injuries happen because people try to do too much too soon. Don't feel bad if you can only do a few reps at first. With each session you'll feel stronger and be able to do more, and by not forcing you'll do your exercises efficiently. A gentle triple slow motion should control the movement.

Read through all the explanations before you start. Of course you won't be able to attain these positions right away, but you'll learn the correct position so you won't be doing the exercises wrong, you'll be protecting your back from unnecessary strain, and your progress will be amazingly fast. Whatever level you work at is the right level for you.

I have designed Callanetics to work your muscles in a certain sequence so they don't become fatigued, and each set complements the one that follows. You should always do these exercises in the exact order shown until your muscles become strong.

Relax Your Entire Body

It is often very hard for me to explain the Callanetics concept of meditation in motion, because what you'll be doing is relaxing *while* you're working the muscle. You don't need to tense up to work and strengthen a muscle effectively. Gentleness is far more productive, and it also means you'll be in control of the motion instead of the motion controlling you. The minimum amount of work will then bring you the maximum effect.

If you are relaxed, you can allow your muscles to work more deeply while you put no strain on your lower back or neck. You'll feel your body literally *melt into the floor, like a rag doll, as light and flowing as a feather.* Think lovely, relaxing thoughts, breathe naturally, and allow yourself to visualize or fantasize about whatever you like. Time will fly by, especially when you see such quick results.

Coming Up Off the Floor

We continually forget to protect and take care of our backs. Getting up properly is so important—but usually we just jerk ourselves instead of rising gracefully in a fluid, easy motion. Here's how you should always do it:

1. Lying on the floor, with your knees bent and relaxed, gently roll your torso and your bent knees over to the right to rest on the floor.

2. Place your hands on the floor, even with your shoulder, supporting most of your weight with your left arm. In triple slow motion, slowly start lifting your body up to a sitting position.

3. Using the strength of your arms, bring yourself up to a kneeling position. In triple slow motion, take either your right or left leg up, bent, until your foot is resting on the floor. Do not lock your elbows.

4. Bring your other leg up. Then tighten your buttocks and curl your pelvis up.

5. Gently, keeping your head down, in triple slow motion, roll up one vertebra at a time until you are in a standing position. Your head comes up last.

Callanetics Basic Routine

If you're already familiar with the Callanetics books, videos, and classes, these exercises will be delightfully familiar. If you're new to Callanetics or any exercise program, you should do a Beginner's routine to ease you into the fabulous world of a tighter, younger figure. Do only the exercises that are starred; I've put in a Beginner's rep count that will be lower than the regular routine. The Beginner's program will only take one half hour, and you should try to do it at least two to three times a week. Once you've mastered it, I hope you progress on to the routines you'll see in the books *Callanetics, Callanetics for Your Back, Super Callanetics,* and *Callanetics Countdown.* If your back bothers you, I urge you to use *Callanetics for Your Back.* You can also use the routines in my videos *Callanetics, Beginning Callanetics, Super Callanetics, Quick Callanetics (Hips, Stomach, Legs),* and *AM/PM Callanetics.*

As always, you *must* consult a medical doctor before beginning any exercise program. *Always work at your own pace.*

Warm-ups (Exercises with an* are for beginners.)

Stretch the Spine—
Loosen the Knees

*Up and Down

1. Stand with your feet hip width apart. Stretch both your arms up to the ceiling as high as you can, and stretch your torso up as well. Tighten your buttocks, and curl your pelvis up. Stretch your torso up even more. Keep your knees relaxed and your feet flat on the floor.

2. In one smooth motion, gently bend your knees as much as you can, and lower your upper body toward the floor, with your arms reaching forward and your torso stretching out and away.

3. Very gently swing your arms back, raising them as high as you can behind your body. Your knees will straighten slightly and your buttocks will rise with the motion of your arms going toward your back and then up.

4. Just as you are about to reverse the movement to return to your upstretched position, tighten your buttocks and curl your pelvis up even

more than you think you can. Keep it curled up until you return to your original starting position, with arms and torso once again stretching up to the ceiling. If you have a swayback, curl your pelvis up as much as you can to stretch your arms and torso up.

Repetitions: Work up to 5

Beginners: 3

Do not arch your back while stretching your arms toward the ceiling.

Do not lock your knees or tense your feet.

Keep your shoulders and neck relaxed.

Stretches the Spine— Loosens the Knees

*Swing

This is basically the same gentle, swinging stretch as Up and Down, except you will stay in a semicrouching position.

1. Stand with your feet hip width apart. Stretch both arms up toward the ceiling. Bend your knees a little. Tighten your buttocks and curl your pelvis up. Now stretch your torso even more. Keep your knees relaxed and your feet flat on the floor. Gently bend your knees as much as you can and lower your upper body toward the floor, your arms reaching forward and aiming toward the floor.

2. From this position gently swing your arms backward and forward. Relax your entire body, as if you were a floppy rag doll, sweeping your arms back and forth as your knees gently move up and down.

3. When you have finished your repetitions, tighten your buttocks and curl your pelvis up. Slowly return to the starting position, rounding your torso up one vertebra at a time, with your head coming up last.

Repetitions: 5

Beginners: 3

Keep your shoulders and knees totally relaxed.

Let go of your neck.

Tightens the underarms— Expands and stretches the chest and spine—Loosens and relieves tension in the neck and between your shoulder blades

*Underarm Tightener

1. Stand erect, with your feet hip width apart. Bend your knees slightly. Take both arms up and out to the sides, keeping them perfectly straight and even with your shoulders. Slowly start rolling your hands forward, thumbs aiming down, then turn your wrists over so that your palms are face up, with your thumbs aiming up toward the ceiling. Now, with your knees still bent slightly, tighten your buttocks and curl your pelvis up even more than you think you can to protect your lower back. Make sure your spine is straight and your head is erect. Raise your shoulders to stretch your spine even more.

2. Gently take your straight arms behind your back as if you're trying to get your shoulder blades to touch. You'll notice your shoulders will drop. Try to keep your hands as high as your shoulders, your arms straight, and your shoulders, head, and torso held erect. Without jerking, slowly move your arms one-quarter to one-half inch closer together in tiny pulsing movements, as if you were trying to get your thumbs to touch each other. Be aware that gravity will keep trying to pull your arms down and your head and shoulders forward.

You may find it difficult to keep your elbows straight at first, but keep trying and eventually you'll get it! When you're finished, bend your elbows and take your arms down in triple slow motion.

Repetitions: 75, working up to 100

Beginners: 25, working up to 100

Keep your pelvis curled up.

Do not allow gravity to pull your arms down. Keep them as high as possible.

Relax your entire body, especially your neck. Keep your shoulders pulled back and relaxed.

Do not lock your knees.

Do not lean your torso, take your head forward, or arch your back. Keep your torso stretched up to the ceiling.

Do not bend your elbows. Keep your wrists turned over and thumb and fingers aimed up to the ceiling.

Stretches the waist, hips, spine, back of shoulders, and underarm area—Reduces the waist

*Waist Away

1. Stand with your feet hip width apart. Put your left hand on or just below your left hip, with your elbow out directly to the side to protect your lower back. Reach your right arm up as high as you can, palm facing inwards. Bend your knees slightly. Tighten your buttocks and curl your pelvis up—try to do it even more than you think you can. Try to reach up even higher to stretch your torso and waist even more.

2. Keeping your right arm stretched and as straight as possible, and with your pelvis still curled up, gently lean and stretch your torso and right arm directly over to your left side as far as you can, without moving your hips or forcing. In triple slow motion, pulse your torso (not your arm) up and down, no more than one-quarter to one-half inch, while stretching your torso and right arm over to the left in a smooth, continuous motion. Keep your neck and left shoulder relaxed.

3. To come out of this stretch, do not stand up straight—that would put pressure on your lower back. Instead, gently bend your knees as much as you can and continue to stretch your right arm over to your left side. In one smooth, continuous motion bring your right arm and torso around to the front, slowly extending them down toward the floor and over to your right side. Feel the lovely stretch in your spine.

4. When your back is totally relaxed and you can't go any farther to the right, slowly come up to your original position by tightening your buttocks, curling up your pelvis, and rounding your torso vertebra by vertebra. Your head comes up last.

Repetitions: 75 on each side, working up to 100

Beginners: 25 on each side, working up to 100

Beginners: If you have a bad back, you can do this exercise while sitting in a chair, keeping your spine straight. To reverse sides or come out of this exercise, slowly lower your arm and straighten your spine, until you have returned to the original position.

Stretches the hamstring muscles, calves, lower back, and the area between your shoulder blades as well as your neck

Standing Hamstring Stretch

1. Stand with feet hip width apart. Bend your knees, and without forcing, very slowly round your torso over in front of you as much as you can, trying to aim your head down between your knees. Keep your body relaxed and your head tucked under. Gently grasp the inside of each calf or ankle with both hands and aim your elbows out to the sides to stretch the area between your shoulder blades. In triple slow motion, pulse your torso one-quarter to one-half inch, trying to ease your head between your legs, without forcing. Do not bounce. Relax your shoulders and neck and let your feet melt into the floor.

2. When you have completed your repetitions, gently move your torso over to your right side. Clasp your right calf or ankle with both hands, your right hand on the inside of your calf or ankle and your left hand on the outside. Keep your elbows aimed out to the sides and your knees bent. Eventually, try to ease your head in between your right arm and right leg as far as it will go without forcing. In triple slow motion, pulse your torso no more than one-quarter to one-half inch.

3. Keeping your knees relaxed, gently move your torso over to your left side, clasping your left calf or ankle with both hands, your left hand on the inside of your ankle or calf and your right hand on the outside. Keep your elbows bent and out to the sides. Try to ease your head between your left arm and left leg, and gently pulse your torso one-quarter to one-half inch.

4. To come out of this stretch, in triple slow motion, gently move your torso and hands back to the center, and with your torso relaxed, let your body and arms hang loosely, as if you were a rag doll. Bend your knees as much as you can, lowering your buttocks toward the floor so you are in a crouching position. Tighten your buttocks, curl your pelvis up, and, with your arms hanging loosely in front, slowly round your torso up, vertebra by vertebra, to return to your original standing position. Gently bring your head up last.

Repetitions: 20 each to the center, right, and left

Do not force.

Do not tense or lock your knees.

Keep your pulses fluid and small. Never jerk or bounce.

If you have sciatica, keep your knees bent at all times. Or try the Lying-Down Hamstring Stretch instead.

Unlocks tension—Loosens the neck and shoulders

*Neck Relaxer

1. Stand erect or sit up straight in a chair, feet hip width apart, knees bent, feet forward. Relax your shoulders, as if they were dripping into the floor. Relax your entire body, without arching your back or sticking out your buttocks.

2. In triple slow motion, stretch your neck up, then lower your chin toward your chest. Relax your jaw and shoulders, keeping your torso erect and your shoulders back.

3. Leading with your chin, gently move your head toward your right shoulder until your nose is even with the middle of your shoulder. Look over your shoulder as far as possible, trying to stretch your neck even more. Hold for a slow count of five.

4. With your neck still stretched, slowly bring your chin down to your chest and move it toward your left shoulder in one continuous slow motion. Look over your left shoulder as much as possible, holding for a slow count of five. Slowly return your head to the center. This sequence counts as 1 repetition.

Repetitions: 5 to each side

Beginners: 2, working up to 5

Do not make any sharp or sudden movements that could injure your neck.

Do not hunch or tense your shoulders, or tense your jaw. Keep your lips slightly parted.

Do not lock your knees.

Do not stick out your buttocks or stomach.

Stomach Exercises

Strengthens your abdominal and pectoral muscles—Stretches your neck and spine

*Bent Knee Reach

1. Lie on the floor, knees bent, feet hip width apart and flat on the floor, and arms by your sides. Relax your shoulders. With your head still on the floor, grasp your inner thighs with all your might. Take your elbows out to the sides as much as you can, and then aim them up toward the ceiling to stretch your upper back muscles.

2. With your lower back relaxed and melting into the floor, slowly round your head and shoulders off the floor, aiming your nose and shoulders in toward your chest. At the same time, take your elbows out and up toward the ceiling even more. You'll still be holding on to your inner thighs.

3. With your head and shoulders rounded as much as possible, take your hands off your thighs and gently lower your arms to the sides of your legs, aiming them straight in front of you, palms down and about six to twelve inches off the floor. In triple slow motion, gently pulse your upper torso (not your head or arms) or lower torso back and forth no more than one-quarter to one-half inch. Totally relax your buttocks and mid to lower back. Try to keep your head and shoulders rounded and aimed in toward your chest as much as you can. Do not force this movement.

4. To come out of this exercise, in triple slow motion, lower your head and shoulders back to the floor, rolling down one vertebra at a time.

Repetitions: 75, working up to 100

Beginners: 25, working up to 75

Really grab your inner thighs when you're rounding up.

Do not tense your stomach muscles—or your legs or body. Relax and let your lower back melt into the floor. Your neck stays very relaxed.

Keep your shoulders rounded in off the floor as much as possible.

Do not jerk or bounce, or rock back and forth. Your arms, shoulders, and neck all move together with your upper torso when you're pulsing.

Do not tense your buttocks. They should not move at all.

Never aim your face toward the ceiling. Always aim your nose and shoulders in toward your rib cage.

Always take a breather whenever you need to. Do not return to the floor—grasp your inner thighs with your hands and hold this rounded position while you rest. Then ease yourself back into position.

Beginners: Keep your bent legs up on a chair or a sofa, especially if you have back problems or until your legs are stronger. If you tend to lift with your neck, cradle it with both hands. Keep your elbows out. Don't allow your back muscles to assist you.

Strengthens your abdominal muscles

*Single Leg Raise

1. Lie on the floor with your knees bent and aiming up toward the ceiling, feet hip width apart and flat on the floor. Bend your right knee in toward your chest as far as you can.

2. Gently raise your right leg straight up, with your toes relaxed and pointing toward the ceiling. If you can't raise your leg straight up or straighten it at first, don't worry. Work at the level that feels comfortable for you.

3. Keeping your head on the floor, with both hands grasp the back of your right thigh, just above your knees. Take both elbows out to the sides as far as they can go, and then aim them up toward the ceiling to stretch the area between your shoulder blades.

4. In triple slow motion, round your head and shoulders off the floor, bringing your head up first and aiming your nose and shoulders in toward your chest. At the same time, take your elbows out to the side and then up even more for a lovely stretch. Always round your head and shoulders more than you think you can. Keep your lower and middle back on the floor. Try to aim your nose in toward your chest even more.

5. When you can't round in any farther, slowly straighten your left leg in front of you, raised no more than a foot off the floor. If that's too difficult at first, either rest your left leg on the floor or return it to the starting position with your knee bent. Take your hands off your legs and place your arms by your sides, extending them straight out in front, palms

down, six inches to one foot off the floor. From this position, in triple slow motion, gently pulse your upper torso—not your head, arms, or lower torso—one-quarter to one-half inch forward and back, allowing your back to melt into the floor.

If you need to take a breather, grasp your uplifted leg just below the knee with both hands, hold your rounded position with your elbows out, and breathe deeply and naturally. You can also bend the other knee and let that foot rest on the floor. To continue, return your left leg to its straightened position, and then take your elbows out and up even more before releasing your hands.

6. To come out of this exercise, in triple slow motion gently bend first your right knee and then your left knee, so both feet are resting on the floor. Slowly lower your head and shoulders back to the floor, rolling down one vertebra at a time.

7. Repeat on the other side.

Repetitions: 75, working up to 100

Beginners: 25, working up to 75

Try not to let your shoulders sink back to the floor as they will tend to do at first. Keep them rounded as much as you can. The more you round, the deeper your stomach muscles will work, producing faster results.

Keep your entire body relaxed. Especially your back; don't let it take over.

Do not lock your knees or tense your legs, stomach muscles, or neck. If you tend to lift with your neck, cradle it with both hands.

Do not tighten your buttocks or stomach muscles.

Never aim your face toward the ceiling—this strains your neck. Always aim your nose in toward your chest.

Take breathers whenever you need to.

Beginners: You can do this exercise with your raised leg resting on a chair or sofa. You can also hold on to your right thigh if you're not feeling quite strong enough yet.

Strengthens your abdominal muscles

Double Leg Raise

1. Lying on the floor, feet hip width apart, bend your knees, one at a time, in toward your chest.

2. Extend your legs, one at a time, up toward the ceiling, with your toes pointed and relaxed. Try to straighten your legs, but don't worry if you have to bend them at first.

3. Grasp your outer thighs with both hands, and aim your elbows out to the sides as much as you can and then up as high as you can. Gently round your head and shoulders off the floor even more than you think you can, aiming your nose and shoulders in toward your chest. At the same time, take your elbows out and up even more.

4. Once you are rounded and in position, let go of your legs and place your arms by your sides, extending them straight out in front, palms down, six inches to one foot off the floor. From this position gently pulse your upper torso—not your head, arms, or lower torso—forward and back, no more than one-quarter to one-half inch.

   If you need to take a breather, grab hold of your outer thighs with both hands, hold your rounded position with your elbows still aimed out to the sides, and breathe deeply and naturally. Or you can bend both knees in toward your chest and roll back down to the floor, one vertebra at a time. Before continuing the count, be sure to return to your original starting position by taking your elbows out and up and rounding your head and shoulders toward your chest.

5. To come out of this exercise, in triple slow motion, gently bend your knees and lower your feet to the floor, one at a time. Then slowly lower your head and shoulders back to the floor, rolling down vertebra by vertebra, totally relaxed.

Repetitions: 50, working up to 100

Aim your elbows out and up as far as they will go.

Keep your head and shoulders rounded and off the floor as much as you can, aiming your nose in toward your chest.

Keep your entire body relaxed. Do not tense your buttocks or stomach muscles.

Let your lower back melt into the floor.

Take breathers whenever you need to.

Leg Exercises

Strengthens and tightens the legs, buttocks, and abdominal muscles— Keeps the pelvis flexible— Stretches the spine and area between the shoulder blades

*Pelvic Wave Leg Strengtheners

1. Stand at your barre, or hold on to a sturdy piece of furniture, with your feet turned out to the sides. Go up on the balls of your feet, heels together, knees bent, and arms straight but relaxed. In triple slow motion, with your torso erect but relaxed and your neck stretched yet relaxed, lower your torso two inches straight down toward the floor, keeping your heels together. Do not arch your back.

2. Tighten your buttocks and curl your pelvis up. Then curl it up again, more than you think you can. Gently release your pelvis without pushing your buttocks back. The more you curl your pelvis up, the more your upper torso will round.

3. In triple slow motion, go down two more inches, tighten your buttocks, and curl your pelvis up even more. Feel the stretch in your spine. Gently release.

4. Go down another two inches, tighten your buttocks, and curl your pelvis up even more. Your inner thighs are really working.

5. Reverse the movement, going up two inches, tightening your buttocks and curling your pelvis up and then releasing each time, in triple slow motion, until you return to the starting position. This entire sequence equals one repetition.

Repetitions:　3, working up to 5 sets

Beginners:　2, working up to 5 sets. Only go up and down twice, not three times, at first.

Hold on tight for extra support—you're working lots of different groups of muscles at once in this exercise!

Do not look down, slump forward, or stick out your behind.

Keep your shoulders and knees relaxed.

Do not allow your buttocks to drop below your knees—this creates too much pressure on your knees.

Strengthens and tightens the leg muscles

Pliés

1. In the same position as the Pelvic Wave, hold your barre or piece of sturdy furniture with both hands, your arms straight and lose. Stand on the balls of your feet with your heels together. Torso erect.

2. In triple slow motion, lower your torso straight down as low as you can. Then, still in triple slow motion, raise yourself back up, breathing normally. This exercise is done in one smooth motion.

Repetitions: Work up to 10

Do not let your heels drop to the floor when coming up.

Do not let your buttocks drop below your knees—this creates too much pressure on your knees.

Do not tense your shoulders, arch your back, or stick out your buttocks. Keep your spine straight and your neck stretched.

The slower you do this Plié and the more erect your torso, the stronger your front thigh muscles will become.

Stretches the neck, spine, between the shoulder blades, buttocks, inner thighs, hamstring muscles, and calves

*Hamstring Stretch #1—Up and Over

1. Standing straight, take your right leg up and rest your heel on your barre or a piece of sturdy furniture. Your left foot should be turned out slightly for balance, with your left knee straight but relaxed.

2. Stretch your torso and arms up toward the ceiling. Turn to the side, stretch up even more, and then turn back to the front. Still stretching up, slowly round your torso over your right leg.

3. When you're over as far as you can go, gently crisscross your hands on your shin or front thigh (not the knee), letting them rest lightly. Take your elbows out to the side. Do not lock your knees.

4. Gently move your torso up and down one-quarter to one-half inch, or just hold the position.

5. To come out of this exercise, walk your hands back up your legs and

gently lower your right leg to the floor in triple slow motion. Repeat on the other side.

Repetitions: Work up to 50

Beginners: Do 10 on each side, working up to 50

Do not do this stretch if you have sciatica.

If resting your heel on the barre or furniture is uncomfortable, place a folded-up towel underneath it.

Keep your hips even. Keep your elbows bent and stretched out. Do not lock your knees.

Do not force your stretch, or bounce.

Beginners: With knee bent you can do this with a barre or piece of furniture level with or lower than your knee. The foot on the floor can be turned out slightly for balance.

Buttocks—Hips—Outer Thighs

Tightens your buttocks ***Bringing Up the Rear—Sitting**

1. Sit on your left buttock in front of your barre or piece of furniture, using a mat or towel as a cushion if you like. Rest your left knee on the floor in front of you, with your left knee bent and aiming outward and your left heel placed eight to ten inches away from the midline of your body. Your right leg is out to the side with the knee bent and your knee in line with your right hip. Your right foot rests on the floor behind you, with toes relaxed and aiming to the back. Both hips face forward.

2. Place your left hand on the barre for support. Making sure that your right hip remains facing the barre, place your right hand on your right hip—not on your upper leg—to roll your right hip forward as much as you can. It will always roll forward more than you think it can. As your hip is rolled forward, your torso automatically turns to the left and your right foot comes up off the floor. If it doesn't, use your right hand to assist it.

3. Place your right hand on the barre and lift your right knee off the floor no more than 3 inches. Keep your right hip rolled forward and your torso straight and relaxed. In triple slow motion, pulse your knee back and forth, no more than one-quarter to one-half inch, and then forward, so your knee is once again in line with your right hip. Try to relax your entire body, even as you hold on tightly to the barre for support.

4. Repeat on the other side.

Repetitions: 75, working up to 100 pulses

Beginners: 20, working up to 100 pulses

If this is too difficult at first, or you feel it in your lower back, lean directly over to the opposite side of the leg you are working; this will enable you to lift your knee off the floor. You can also rest your left hand on the floor to support your torso, or bring your working knee forward a little.

Do not take your torso forward or push your stomach out, as this strains your lower back. Keep it erect. Do not arch your lower back. Keep your hips even.

Once you have lifted your knee off the floor and started your pulses, do not move your hip. Only your leg moves back and forth. Keep your leg relaxed.

Do not tense your neck or hunch your shoulders.

Work at your own pace. Relax into the floor and take frequent breathers, especially if your foot starts to feel heavy and dragging down.

Tightens your buttocks ***Out to the Side—Sitting**

1. Start in the same position as the Bringing Up the Rear—Sitting (p. 144), with your left leg bent and resting on the floor in front of you. Extend your right leg straight out to the side of your body so that your toes are even with your right hip, and place your left hand on your barre or piece of heavy furniture. Place your right hand on your right hip and slowly roll that hip and leg over so that the tops of your toes are trying to aim into the floor. Bend your knee if you need to.

2. Place your right hand on your barre and then pull your right leg in toward your body, letting your torso lean over directly to your left side if necessary.

3. Lift your right foot off the floor no more than 3 inches, and gently pulse it up and down, no more than one-quarter to one-half inch. The movement remains so small because your hip has been rolled forward so much.

4. Repeat on the other side.

Repetitions: 75, working up to 100

Beginners: 20, working up to 100

You can brace yourself on the floor or sofa if you need more support. Or lean over to the opposite side of your working leg, making sure that your lower back stays stretched.

When rolling your hip forward, do not allow your torso or stomach to push forward—this strains your lower back. Keep your torso erect yet relaxed. Never arch your back.

Lift your leg from the foot, not the hip. Don't raise it too high. Your hips do not move up and down at all as you pulse. Keep your working hip forward as much as you can; don't let it roll back. Keep your hips even.

Totally relax your body, especially your shoulders and neck.

Work at your own pace, and take breathers whenever you need to.

Keep your shoulders relaxed.

The Entire Body

For greater strength, energy, and vitality— Strengthens the stomach and thigh muscles

Open and Close

*Do not do this exercise if you are pregnant.
1. Sit on the floor with your upper back against your barre or a sturdy piece of furniture, and hold on to the top of it as if there were a barre above your head. Bend your knees and take them in toward your chest.

Point your toes. Scoot your buttocks forward four to five inches away from the furniture so you won't be sitting on your tailbone, to take pressure off your lower back. As you scoot forward, try to get the bottom of your buttocks to round up and in toward your navel—similar to a pelvic curl-up without tightening your buttocks. Gently drop your chin to stretch your spine even more.

2. Clasping the barre firmly with both hands, relax your shoulders and neck. Without locking your knees, slowly straighten your legs, raising them as high as you can without forcing, pointing your toes up toward the ceiling. You are now sitting in a jackknife position. In triple slow motion, open your legs as wide as you can, then close them.

3. To come out of this exercise, gently bring your legs to the closed position and bend your knees, bringing your knees in close to your chest. Slowly lower your legs to the floor.

Repetitions: 2 sets of 5, working up to 4 sets of 5

Make sure your barre or piece of furniture is strong enough to hold your weight.

If you can't lift your legs at first, don't worry—simply straighten them out on the floor. As you get stronger you'll be able to lift them.

Relax your legs, especially your knees. Although your toes are pointed, keep your feet relaxed.

Never force your legs farther apart than they can comfortably go.

Keep your chin down.

Take as many breathers as you need to.

Stretches

Stretches the inner thighs, spine, neck, underarms, legs

*Inner Thigh Stretch—Sitting

1. Sitting on the floor, spread your legs as far apart as they can go without forcing. Rest your palms on either the floor in front of you, or on

your thighs. Gently push your pubic bone into the floor, and then scoot it forward a tiny bit for a better stretch. Stretch your torso up, then take your elbows out to the side and around your upper back. Relax your shoulders and your neck. In triple slow motion, round your upper back forward and down until your head and shoulders are down toward the floor as far as they can go without straining. Relax your body, and feel the lovely stretch in your lower back and inner thighs. With your head, neck, and shoulders working together as a unit, gently pulse your torso one-quarter to one-half inch, up and down. Do not bounce.

2. When you've finished your repetitions, slowly walk your hands across the floor to the right, and move your torso over to your right leg. Gently crisscross your hands on your leg or wherever is comfortable (but not on your knee), and aim your elbows out to the sides. Almost imperceptibly, pulse your torso toward your feet, one-quarter to one-half inch, aiming your head down toward your leg to stretch your neck. Eventually you'll be aiming to rest your head on your legs.

3. Next go over to the left. Slowly walk your hands across the floor, moving your torso over to your left leg. Gently crisscross your hands on your leg, aiming your elbows out, and repeat the tiny, pulsing movements. Relax your entire body, melting into the floor.

4. To come out of this stretch, gently walk your hands back to the center. Walk them back up, slowly straightening your torso, one vertebra at a time, to return to your original sitting position.

Repetitions: 50 pulses to center, right, and left

Beginners: 10 pulses each way, working up to 50

If you have sciatica, always keep your knees bent during this exercise.

Do not force or bounce your body down.

Keep your entire body relaxed. Do not lock your knees.

Beginners: Bend your knees as much as you have to, and place your hands on your upper thighs, aiming your elbows out to the sides. Do your delicate pulses from this position. Stay relaxed.

Stretches the neck, spine, area between the shoulder blades, inner thighs, and backs of legs—Strengthens the pectoral muscles

*Hamstring Stretch—Sitting

1. Sit on the floor with your shoulders erect, legs together in front of you, toes pointed yet relaxed. Rest your hands on the front of your thighs and aim your elbows out to the sides to stretch the area between your shoulder blades. Stretch your torso up. Now, very gently, round your head and shoulders, aiming your nose and shoulders toward the top of your legs. Keep curling your upper torso until your head and shoulders are rounded as much as possible, without forcing. You will eventually be aiming to rest your head on your legs. Totally relax your body, letting it melt into the floor. Feel the lovely stretch in your lower back and hamstring muscles. Gently pulse your upper torso up and down, no more than one-quarter to one-half inch. Keep your elbows relaxed and out to the sides.

2. To come out of this stretch, slowly walk your hands back up your legs and gently straighten your upper torso, one vertebra at a time, until you are sitting erect. Bring your head up in triple slow motion, last of all.

Repetitions: 50 pulses
Beginners: 20 pulses

If you have sciatica, always keep your knees bent during this exercise.

Don't worry if you can't straighten your legs completely at first. Keep your knees bent until you get stronger.

Keep your upper torso rounded as you go down. Do not force your body down.

Do not bounce or jerk, or pull forward with your neck.

Your entire body is relaxed.

Stretches the inner thighs, backs of the legs, neck, spine, and area between the shoulder blades— Strengthens the pectoral muscles

*Hamstring Stretch—Lying Down

1. Lie on your back, with your knees bent and feet hip width apart. Try to flatten the back of your neck on the floor. Bend your right knee up in toward your chest, and then slowly straighten the leg as much as you can, aiming it upward, without forcing. Don't worry if you can't straighten your leg at first. Clasp your hands behind your right thigh, just above the knee. Move your elbows out to stretch the area between

your shoulder blades, and gently bring your leg as close to your body as you can. In triple slow motion, move your right leg toward you and then back, pulsing no more than one-quarter to one-half inch. Always keep your elbows out, and very relaxed.

2. To protect your back when coming out of this stretch, or when switching sides to work the other leg, release your arms and, in triple slow motion, bring your right knee in toward your chest and place your foot flat on the floor.

3. Repeat on the other side.

Repetitions: 50 to each side

Beginners: 20, working up to 50

If you have sciatica, always keep your knees bent during this exercise.

Do not force your leg up higher than it can go. Do not lock your knees.

Keep the grasp on your thigh, calf, or ankle very loose and relaxed.

Keep your elbows out.

Your entire body is wonderfully relaxed.

Beginners: If this is too difficult at first, simply hold your leg in the raised position for a count of 20 to 50, without pulsing.

Stretches the entire back, spine, area between the shoulder blades, pectorals, buttocks, hips, and outer thighs

*Spine Stretch

1. Lying on the floor, with knees bent and feet flat on the floor, extend your arms out at shoulder level, elbows bent up at right angles, so that the backs of your hands rest on the floor. Your wrists might not touch the floor, but your elbows should always remain on the floor; they will be even with your shoulders. Gently bring your right knee up to your chest. Let your left leg gently ease down so that it is fully extended and resting on the floor.

2. Keeping both elbows on the floor, move your bent right knee over to your left side, away from your body as much as you can. In triple slow motion, pulse your left knee and leg up and down, one-quarter to one-half inch.

3. Keep your entire body relaxed; do not force your knee farther down than it can go. When you have become more stretched, gravity will bring your right foot and then your right knee nearer to the ground. Eventually your foot and then your knee will be resting on the floor.

4. To go over to the other side, in triple slow motion, keeping your right knee bent, bring it back to your chest and then place your right foot on the floor with your knee still bent. Bend your left knee into your chest, and then slide your right foot down to the floor. This is all done in one smooth, continuous motion.

5. Repeat this stretch on the opposite side.

6. To come out of this stretch, in triple slow motion, keeping your knee bent, bring it to your chest, and then place your foot on the floor. Bend your other knee, and place that foot flat on the floor. Then ease yourself up to a standing position by rolling over to your side and slowly going up by gently using your arms.

Repetitions: Work up to 50 pulses on each side

Beginners: 20, working up to 50 pulses on each side

Do not force your bent leg down to the floor.

Do not lift your shoulders or elbows off the floor.

No forcing. Gravity is helping you here.

Keep your entire body relaxed, especially your neck.

Pelvis—Front and Inner Thighs

Strengthens the buttocks, thighs, lower back, stomach, feet, and pelvic muscles—Stretches the arms and spine— Loosens the pelvic area

*Pelvic Rotations

1. Sit on your heels, with your torso erect. Use a mat or towel to cushion your feet and knees. Keep your knees together and your legs relaxed. Stretch your arms up over your head and clasp your hands together. Stretch your torso up and feel the stretch in your stomach and back.

2. Lift your buttocks up three inches off your heels. Gently move your right hip over to the right side as far as you can.

3. Tighten your buttocks and curl your pelvis up. At the same time, roll your pelvis forward, to the front, aiming it up and in toward your navel. Release your pelvis as you move your left hip over to the left side as far as you can. Then move your buttocks to the back, completing the circle. One complete circle counts as one repetition.

4. Working at your own pace, complete the repetitions to this side, moving in triple slow motion, as you circle to the right, front, left, and back. Take a breather for a few seconds, then lift yourself back into position, feeling the stretch in your lower back.

5. Repeat starting to the left.

Repetitions: 5 rotations in each direction, working up to 10

Beginners: 2 rotations in each direction, working up to 10

If you have bad knees, you can do this in a chair. Lift your body up with your arms. Or try it standing up, with knees bent and feet hip width apart and facing forward.

If your calves bother you, lean your torso forward to take the pressure off. Hold on to one side of a sofa if you need to for balance. You can also spread your knees slightly farther apart.

Keep your entire body relaxed.

The more you can curl your pelvis up and in toward your navel when rolling your pelvis forward, the more effective this exercise will be.

Don't lean forward or stick out your stomach.

The entire movement should be one smooth, flowing circle—hip—pelvis—hip—behind. Only your pelvis moves. Visualize your pelvis rotating in a large circle in triple slow motion.

Strengthens the leg muscles, stomach, buttocks, and calves— Stretches the spine

Pelvic Scoop

1. Kneel on a mat, knees together, with your feet behind you and your legs relaxed. Keep your arms and shoulders relaxed and your spine straight. Lift your arms up and over your head, stretching as high as you possibly can, and clasp your hands together. Feel the stretch in your lower back. Lower your arms about a foot in front of you, and round your upper torso forward as if you were diving into a pool.

2. Keeping your spine straight, aim your buttocks toward the back, at the same time aiming them down toward your heels and still feeling the stretch in your spine. Do not simply sit down on your heels, and do not arch your back.

3. When you have stretched your buttocks to the point where they are delicately brushing your heels, gently tighten your buttocks, and then curl up your pelvis even more than you think you can, in a slow, scooping motion. (Your ability to curl up regulates the intensity of this exercise.) Hold for a split second and, if you can, raise your arms back up until your hands are above your head in the starting position. Then keep curling your pelvis up, and use the strength of your thighs to lift your body back up to the original kneeling position. When your pelvis is curled up, your buttocks will be farther from your heels.

Repetitions: Work up to 5

Keep your pelvis curled up and your buttocks tightened when you are returning to your original kneeling position.

Do not arch your back when aiming your buttocks to the back and down toward your heels. You will not be just sitting straight down and then going back up again!

Try not to put pressure on your calves. Take your arms and torso forward if necessary to release them.

Take a breather if you need one.

Keep your entire body relaxed.

You can do this standing.

Stretches the neck, pectoral muscles, spine, and thighs—Strengthens the buttocks, inner thighs, and stomach

*Front Thigh Stretch

1. Sit on your heels, with your knees together and feet relaxed. Use a pillow or mat to cushion your legs from knee to toe, if you like. Relax your shoulders. Lean back, resting your weight on your heels and placing your palms on the floor behind you, with fingers facing away from your body. Relax your neck. Still sitting on your heels, tighten your buttocks and curl your pelvis up, aiming it in toward your navel, then curl it up even more.

2. Lift your buttocks up off your heels no more than one inch. Curl your pelvis up even higher. In triple slow motion, gently pulse your pelvis up and down, still aiming it toward your navel, no more than one-quarter to one-half inch.

3. When you have completed your pulses, relax your buttocks and slowly return to the starting position, sitting on your heels. Relax your entire body.

Repetitions: 10 pulses, working up to 20

Beginners: 10 pulses

Keep your spine straight and do not arch your back.

Do not allow your head to drop back. Do not move your head up and down.

Keep your arms straight but relaxed. Do not put too much pressure on your hands or lock your elbows.

Keep your knees together and your entire body relaxed.

Do not forget to curl your pelvis up. The more the curl, the better the stretch.

Beginners: You can brace yourself against the back of a chair, or on the arms of a sturdy sofa. Keep your knees farther apart if that makes you feel more comfortable. If this stretches your thighs too much, drop your behind down a bit.

You can also do this stretch while standing. Here's how:
1. Stand facing a wall, door, or other stable surface, and rest left hand on it for balance. Bend both knees.

2. Raise your bent right leg, and with foot facing back, grasp your right foot with your right hand. Tighten your buttocks and curl your pelvis up. Pull your leg to the back, feeling the stretch in your front thigh. Hold for a count of 15 to 30.

3. Gently return your leg to the floor. Repeat with your other leg.

Do not place your heel on your buttocks, arch your back, lock your knees, or pull your leg to the side.

Tightens the inner thighs—Stretches the spine—Strengthens the stomach, calves, and feet

*Inner Thigh Squeeze

1. Facing a very sturdy piece of furniture like a stool, chair, table, or desk legs, sit on the floor, with your back straight, your hands resting on the floor by your sides. Bend your knees and place the arch of each foot around the outsides of the stool or table legs so that the toes of each foot are pointing toward each other. Straighten your legs, then gently round your upper torso so that you won't put pressure on your lower back. Gently stretch the back of your neck by letting your head aim down toward your chest.

2. Keeping your toes pointed and relaxed, squeeze your legs as much as you can, as if trying to bring the legs of the stool together. Squeeze for the count, if you can, then relax. Try to squeeze continuously for better results. Your inner thighs are doing all the work.

Repetitions: 75, working up to 100

Beginners: 25, working up to 100

Keep your neck and shoulders, arms and hands relaxed and comfortable.

Do not tense your lower back, or your feet.

Do not lean backward. Keep your upper torso rounded.

Keep your body relaxed at all times.

Take frequent breathers if you need to.

Beginners: Bend your knees at first until you feel stronger. Then you can straighten your legs. If you sit at your desk a lot, this is a good exercise to do there. Place your knees on the outer legs of a table or even a strong trash can, and squeeze!

CHAPTER # CARDIOCALLANETICS

About CardioCallanetics

CardioCallanetics is not your traditional exercise routine. It looks like no other and feels like no other. It was designed specifically to prepare all of us for the physiological and psychological demands of everyday life. Based on simple and fluid ballet and yoga movements that are very easy to follow, CardioCallanetics has no jarring and pounding moves. The workout is rhythmic, soothing, and flowing—yet this exciting new aerobic alternative is challenging to people of all fitness levels. The cardio section is wonderful for pregnant women and older people. You'll learn to develop stamina, maintain your cardiovascular health, reduce stress, burn fat, and invigorate all your senses.

A CardioCallanetics workout lasts one hour: the first half hour is low-impact cardiovascular exercise consisting of a five-to-ten-minute warm-up and stretch, a fifteen-to-twenty-minute low-impact aerobic section, and about a five-minute cooldown and flexibility section; the second half-hour is a traditional Callanetics routine. Together you'll get a perfect balance of aerobic exercise, with muscle strength training, and flexibility and stretching exercises. You'll be working your heart, mind, and body. All you need is a comfortable leotard and tights so you can see your body alignment, and athletic socks or ballet shoes. (You don't need to spend a lot of money on aerobic shoes because you won't be wearing any shoes! So if you work out at home, be sure to do so on a carpeted surface for cushioning.) If you prefer, you can wear a T-shirt and shorts, but it's best if they are made of cotton or one of the special fabrics that wick moisture away from your body, so you don't get overheated.

The CardioCallanetics portion of this workout is aerobic. Here are tips to make your CardioCallanetics experience much more pleasurable:

1. How often should you do CardioCallanetics? To maintain your current fitness level, you should work out two times a week. To improve your fitness level, you must work out three to five times a week.

    *If you wake up one morning feeling "out of it," take your pulse. (You should always know what your resting heart rate is, anyway.) If your resting heart rate is elevated by 10 percent, be very careful not to overexert yourself when you're working out. If your resting heart rate is elevated by 20 percent or more, I don't think you should work out that day. You might be fighting off the flu or a cold, repairing some other injury to your body, or just under a lot of stress.

2. Some dedicated Callanetics students may see themselves as "advanced" because they are extremely skilled at traditional Callanetics. It is very important to remember that traditional Callanetics trains your body for muscle strength through particular moves using very particular motions. CardioCallanetics will be using other moves as well—you'll notice this in the exercise descriptions—so you may have to concentrate on learning this new routine in a very different way at first. Once you get used to the routine, I'm sure you will quickly become accustomed to these movements.

    Do not risk injury by trying to do too much too soon, no matter what exercise routine you follow!

3. Because a full CardioCallanetics class is sixty minutes long, during the half hour of the Cardio portion, feel free to take a water break. Your body must be hydrated before, during, and after each Cardio workout. This is critical for optimal health and to maximize your workout potential. Whenever you do aerobic exercises, you automatically lose fluid from your skin and lungs. A person is already 1 percent dehydrated when she feels "thirsty." By the time there is a 2 percent drop in hydration there is a 10 percent drop in athletic performance; with a 5 percent drop in hydration, there's a 30 *percent* drop in performance. In other words: If you're dehydrated, you are more prone to injury because your body is functioning less efficiently.

So drink up! It's recommended that you drink at least eight to ten cups of water each day. Two hours before a CardioCallanetics class, drink two to three cups of water. Drink at least one cup of water right before class, and one cup after the Cardio workout. Try to avoid a lot of caffeine or any alcohol, as they both add to increased urine production and dehydration.

4. When beginning CardioCallanetics, you may feel a little warmer and a bit more red in the face than you did in a traditional Callanetics program. That's because you'll be sweating—which is great. Not only is sweat a by-product of fat burning so that you sweat more whenever you're expending calories, but it is your body's very efficient mechanism for cooling you down. And when your face gets red, all that means is that your body is circulating more blood to the surface to help you stay cool, and it's wonderful for your complexion.

    When you're fit, your body acclimates itself to dissipating the heat of an exercise session more efficiently, burns fat more efficiently, and maintains a lower heart rate.

5. If you're older or not used to a cardiovascular, aerobic workout, be sensible when you begin this new exercise routine. You'll need a longer warm-up period so your points are lubricated properly, preventing injuries. You might not have as great a range of motion as younger students. You might not be used to breathing harder when you work out. Moderate exercise for an older adult or someone who's not used to working out is equivalent to vigorous exercise for a person who's younger or more fit. Don't worry! Start slowly, and stay at the lower end of your target heart zone (see chapter 2). The more you work out, the easier it becomes. In the Callanetics studio a talk test is used. If you can speak out loud during the Cardio portion, you're doing fine. This is what is referred to as "Listen to your body." Taking an exact pulse is not necessary.

    If you ever feel out of breath, exhausted, or dizzy, *stop* and *take a breather*. An easy way to slow down your workout is to take smaller steps and either lessen your arm movements or cut them out altogether. It's more important to keep your feet moving than to worry about coordinating your arms. As with your breathing, the more you do this routine and become familiar with the step patterns, the easier it will be to add the arm movements.

6. Approximately 85 percent of your workout comes from your leg movements, and only about 10 to 15 percent comes from your arms. This

means that following the leg patterns is the most important aspect of this routine to concentrate upon. First begin with the basic leg patterns, and then build upon them. Once you've gotten the footwork down, add the arm movements.

Your posture should always be lifted—pretend you are stretching your spine two inches higher—as if your energy is radiating up and out through the top of your head.

7. When you're doing your Callanetics exercises during the second half of this workout, you are really going to feel them! *Always work at your own pace.* Whenever you need to, *take a breather,* even if you need it more than usual. If the amount of repetitions is simply too much for you at first, then see that figure as a goal to work up to, and you'll be there sooner than you expected.

Have fun!

The CardioCallanetics Workout:

Cardio Portion–Half an hour

Cardio Warm-up–5 minutes

Remember: These are fluid movements. Do not stop and freeze in the positions indicated in the photographs.

1. Cleansing Breath —
Repetitions: Do 8.

1. Knees bent slightly, with your feet hip width apart, bring your arms down in front of your body and exhale.

2. Begin to bring your arms up and stretch them out to your sides while inhaling.

(continued on next page)

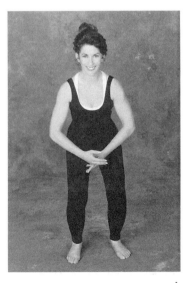

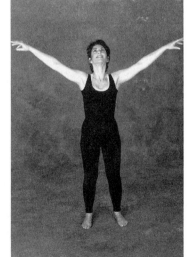

1.

2.

3. Still inhaling, bring your arms up to form a peak above your head, making sure not to extend your arms directly over the top of your head. Do not arch your back. If you feel your back is starting to arch anyway, bring your arms up no farther than your forehead.

4. Bring your arms down in front of your body in the "open pray" position as shown here, palms facing but not touching. Try to pull your energy down to root in your feet and exhale.

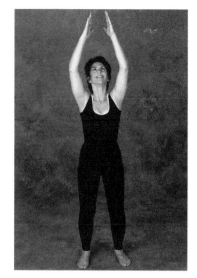

3.

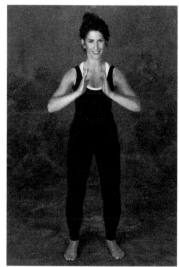

4.

2. Warm-up Swing Lift — *Repetitions: Perform 8 repetitions or as many as needed until the body feels supple and slightly warm.*

1. Stand straight, feet hip width apart. Extend your arms straight out in front of you and then slowly raise them up in a comfortable stretch. Keep your body relaxed. Inhale.

2. Bending your knees, let your arms drop down perpendicular with your shoulders. Look forward, so that your neck will not arch backward. Slowly start to exhale.

(continued on next page)

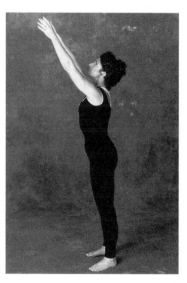

1.

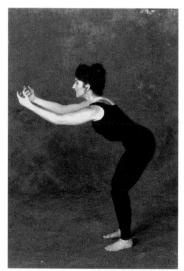

2.

3. Bending your torso forward, swing your arms fully behind you (if possible). Keep your head up so that you can still see in front of you. Be careful not to arch the head up too far. Also, be sure not to bend forward beyond your personal comfort zone. Unsupported forward flexion is not recommended.

4. Return to the starting position by lifting (swinging) your arms over your head, palms facing each other. Inhale on the return up. Exhale slowly.

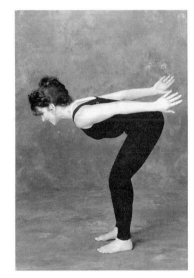

3.

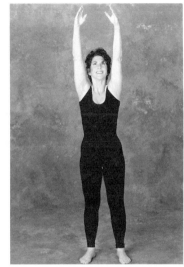

4.

3. Side Circles — *Repetitions: Perform 8 repetitions or as long as is comfortable and warms the body fully. Be sure to repeat this exercise evenly on both sides.*

1. Stand straight, feet hip width apart. Reach your arms up toward the ceiling making sure that the arms are coming toward your eyebrows or forehead and not reaching straight up from the top of your head. This will protect the back from over-arching.

2. Step with your left foot out to the side. Your right leg is nearly straight with a soft knee. Drop your arms down to the right, pulling them across the body in an arc or beginning of a circle.

(continued on next page)

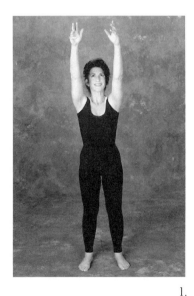

1.

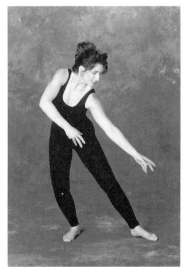

2.

3. Sweep your arms down past your knees and then circle them up toward your right side. They are now extending out to your right side. Keep your elbows and fingers relaxed.

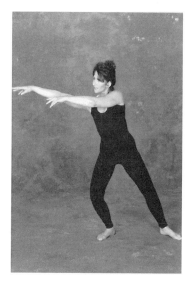

3.

4. Begin to extend your arms up toward the ceiling. Your feet are melting into the floor.

5. Complete the circle sweep by stepping with your left foot back to the starting position. Your arms are now up over your head.

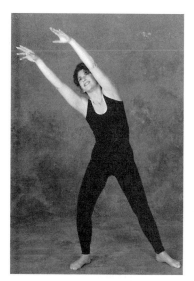

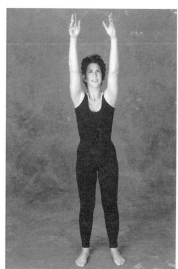

4.

5.

4. Hamstring Stretch — *Repetitions: Hold for at least 30 seconds on each side.*

1. With your feet close together (but not touching), bring your arms up over your head, framing your face. Your elbows are slightly bent and the fingertips of your left hand are about six inches apart from the fingertips of your right hand. Keep your shoulders down and relaxed.

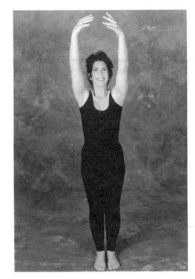

1.

2. Turn your right foot out in a comfortable position. Do not force the angle of your foot to your ankle. Keep your heel down.

3. Step back with your turned-out foot.

(continued on next page)

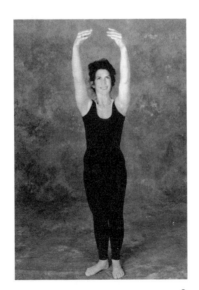

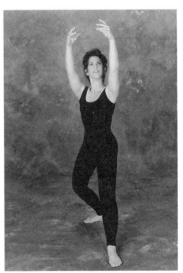

2.

3.

4. Drop your right hand down to rest comfortably on your right thigh. This will help to support your back. Your left arm is still up and extended comfortably.

5. Lean forward and bend your left elbow, bringing your left arm down and behind your back. Raise your left toes, keeping your heel comfortably on the floor. Feel the lovely stretch in your legs. Keep your head up, eyes forward, and your shoulders up and open. Your entire body is relaxed.

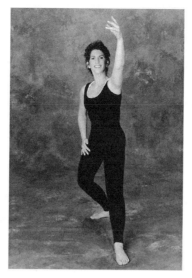

4.

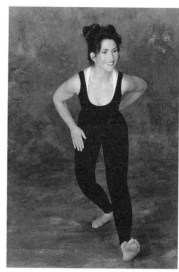

5.

5. Soleus Stretch with Arm Circles — *Repetitions: Hold for at least 30 seconds on each side. Try to hold for up to 90 seconds.*

1. Stand straight, feet hip width apart. Extend your arms straight out in front of you and then slowly raise them up to shoulder level in an easy stretch. Keep your body relaxed. Now step back with your right leg with toes facing forward. Your weight is comfortably balanced. Now bend your right knee a little bit more just until you feel the lovely stretch in your soleus—that is the muscle between your calf and the Achilles tendon just above your heel.

(continued on next page)

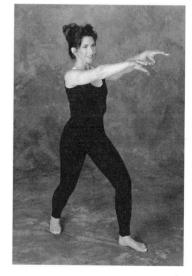

1.

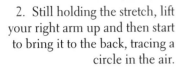

2. Still holding the stretch, lift your right arm up and then start to bring it to the back, tracing a circle in the air.

3. Continue the circle, pulling your right arm behind your body. Only your upper body is moving. Your feet are melting into the floor.

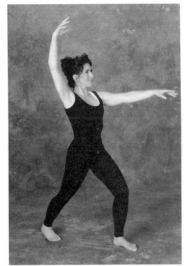

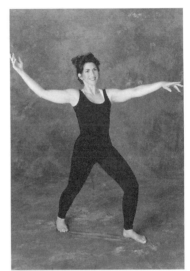

2.

3.

4. Now, as if you were doing the backstroke, circle both your arms backward one at a time. As one falls, bring the other one up in a circle.

5. To finish this stretch, if you like, you can turn your torso slightly to the side, rotating around with your arms still out-stretched at shoulder height. Breathe deeply. Feel how this opens up your entire chest.

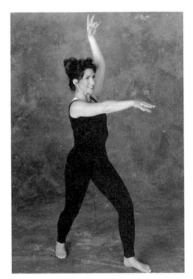

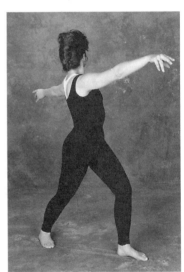

4.

5.

6. Hip Flexor Stretch with Arm Waves — *Repetitions: Hold the stretch for at least 30–90 seconds on each side. Wave your arms up and down at least 8 times during the stretch.*

1. Stand straight, feet hip width apart. Extend your arms straight out in front of you and then slowly raise them up to shoulder level in an easy stretch. Your wrists are loose and palms are facing down. Keep your body relaxed. Now step back with your right leg. Your weight is comfortably balanced. Now bend your right knee a little bit more, just until you feel the same stretch in your soleus.

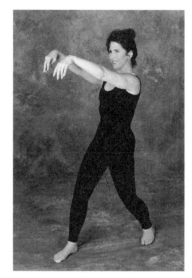

1.

2. With your right knee still bent, press your hip forward very slightly. This will stretch the front of your hip, which is called the hip flexor.

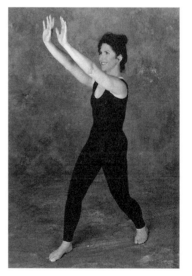

(continued on next page)

2.

3-4-5. Hold the stretch for at least thirty seconds. While in this lovely stretch, wave your arms up and down slowly. Alternate flexing and extending your wrists, as you see here. Keep your wrists and shoulders very relaxed.

6. Repeat other side.

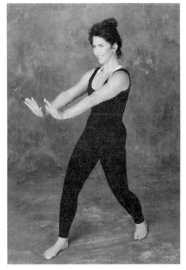

3.

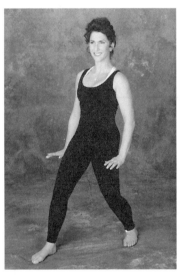

4.

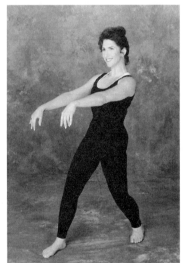

5.

7. Modified Yoga Lean — *Repetitions: Hold for at least 30 seconds on each side*

1. Spread your legs out slightly, a little wider than shoulder width apart. Lean your body over to the right side, sliding your right hand down your leg so that it is supporting your body just above the knee. Do not lean over farther than feels comfortable. Raise your left hand above your shoulder, stretching gently up toward the ceiling with your palm facing forward. Keep your shoulders back and relaxed. You'll feel your chest begin to open up as your body stretches sideways.

2. Come back to the center, then repeat the stretch on the left side.

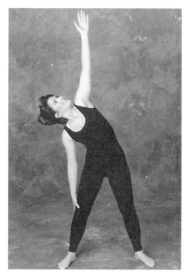

1.

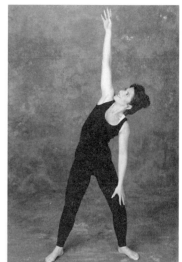

2.

Six Cardio Movements (17 minutes)

8. Step Touch — *Repetitions: Repeat for at least 2–3 minutes.*

Exercise focus: The step-touch is an excellent way to warm up the body before you begin strenuous cardiovascular "aerobic" work.

1. Begin with your feet hip width apart, your knees bent, your arms relaxed at your sides, and wrists bent slightly to curve your hands in front of your hips. Extend your left leg to that you can take a step to the side. This is Count 1.

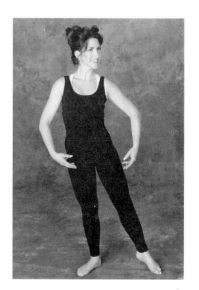

(continued on next page)

1.

2. Extend your left arm out from the shoulder in a "ballet" arm. Make sure that your left hand remains slightly lower than your shoulder, so you won't be putting any stress on your shoulder joint.

3. Perform a "side-step"; this is Count 2. To do this, point your left foot to the side, transfer your weight to your left foot and take a step to the side (to your left). Bring your right leg in to touch your left foot. After the side-step is complete, return to the starting position on the other side.

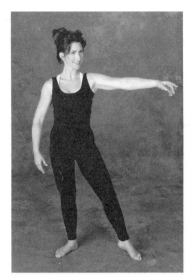

2.

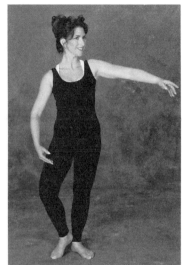

3.

4. Now repeat this step-touch with your right leg extended. This would be Count 3, and 4 would be the beginning position. If you like, you can vary your arm moves. Remember to relax your arms if you feel tired or lose your count.

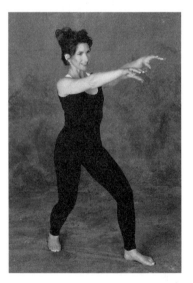

4.

9. Plié Leg Lift — *Repetitions: Perform this exercise for 2 to 3 minutes, taking breaks or lowering arms when necessary.*

Exercise focus: The Plié Leg Lift is performed slowly and therefore is very cardiovascularly and musculoskeletally demanding. This exercise requires control and strength; be sure to take breaks when necessary.

1. This exercise is performed twice as slowly as the step-touch. This makes for a much more demanding exercise. Begin in a plié position.

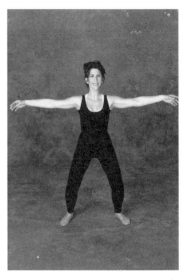

1.

2. Similar to the step-touch, step out with the left foot, transferring your weight to the left. Keep the arms relaxed. These are Counts 1 and 2.

3. While the weight is on the left foot, lift your right leg up a few inches and cross it slightly in front of your body. These are counts 3 and 4. The higher you lift your leg, the more strenuous the exercise. At the same time, lift your left arm. Arm movements make this exercise more demanding. Be sure to stabilize your body by contracting your stomach muscles.

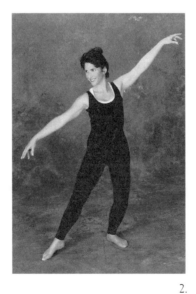

2.

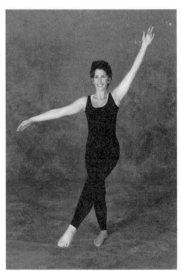

3.

(continued on next page)

4. Place your left leg down and out to the side in a comfortable position. These are Counts 5 and 6. Control this movement by again contracting the stomach muscles and performing the action slowly.

5. Go back to your beginning plié position. These are counts 7 and 8. If you like, you can circle your right arm in front of your body; this may help you maintain the fluid and controlled nature of this exercise.

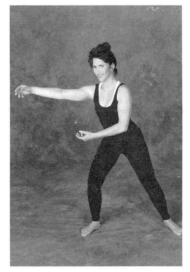

4.

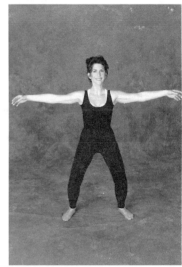

5.

10. Cross Waltz — *Repetitions: Perform this exercise for 2 to 3 minutes.*

Exercise focus: This exercise is smooth and relaxing. To make the exercise harder you can perform the exercises with the larger leg and/or arm movements. Increasing the range of motion will also increase energy expenditure. Smaller movement will decrease energy expenditure.

1. Step with your right foot across your body. Your left leg is extended out slightly to the side with your toes pointed. Gently let your arms follow your legs and cross around your body. This is Count 1.

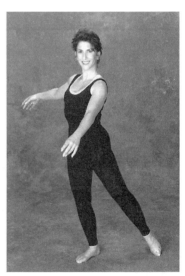

(continued on next page)

1.

2. Lift the back leg and let the right arm swing around the body in a circular motion. This is Count 2.

3. Transfer the weight from your right to your left leg by stepping back on the left foot. Lift the right arm in a smooth arc. This fluid motion completes the movement. This is Count 3.

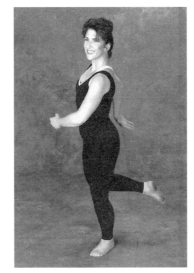 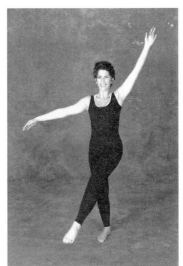

2.   3

4. Return to the plié position and then repeat to the other side. This is count 4.

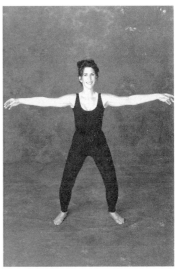

4.

11. Waltz Pull — *Repetitions: Perform this exercise for 2–3 minutes.*

Exercise focus: This dramatic exercise stretches the body and increases the heart rate, encouraging energy expenditure and fat burning.

1. Cross your left foot in front of your right foot, keeping your arms relaxed in a soft ballet arm and your knees bent. This is Count 1.

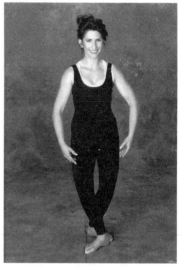

1.

2. Transferring your weight to the right side, pull the body sideways. This is Count 2.

3. Begin to lift your right arm and arc the body around the momentum of the movement. Shift your full body weight to the right leg lifting the arm and feel the full body stretch. This is Count 3. For variation you may lift the inside leg (the left leg).

(continued on next page)

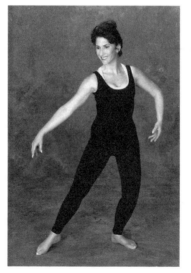

2.

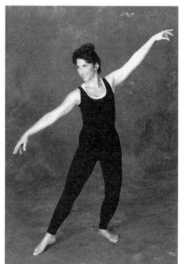

3.

4. Reverse the entire exercise to the other side by reversing the movements. Count 4, return the body back to the beginning position for the opposite side.

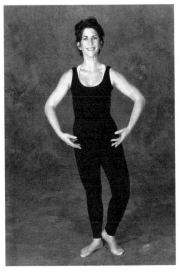

1.

12. Waltz Pull Forward — *Repetitions: Perform this exercise for 2 to 3 minutes.*

Exercise focus: This variation on the Waltz Pull shows how by varying the angle and the range of motion for an exercise the energy expenditure can be increased. This exercise will be slightly more difficult than the traditional Waltz Pull, as shown above, but adds creativity and increases the effort.

1. Relax your arms and keep your knees slightly soft.

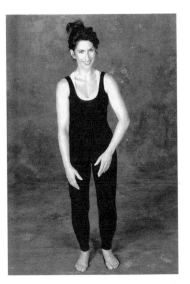

(continued on next page)

1.

2. Step to the side with the right foot reaching forward and to the right with both arms. This is Count 1. When you finish this upward arc motion your arms will be extended in front of you and slightly to the right.

3. Lift your right leg up behind you. These are Counts 2 and 3. This is called a rear extension and will contract your gluteal muscles. At the same time, the arms are lifted in front of you and the back is not arched. Your abdominals must be contracted to support your back.

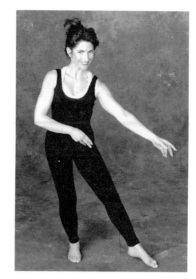

2.

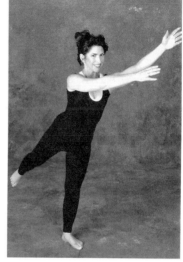

3.

4. To reverse this exercise to the other side, step back with the left foot and pull the right foot in, in front of the left foot. Let the arms relax down by your sides and center the body in a soft plié. This is Count 4.

5. Then begin the exercise to the other side by extending the left arm to the side and the left leg to the side.

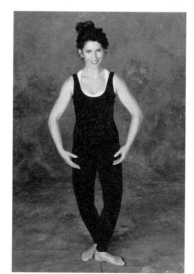

4.

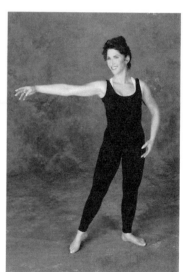

5.

Barre Movements   (3 minutes)—Cool Down

13. Plié at the Barre — *Repetitions: Repeat the entire 8-Count combination 8 times, and then repeat on the other side.*

Exercise focus:

Do this sequence very slowly and with as much control as possible. It will start to slow down your heart rate.

1. With your right arm braced against your barre or sturdy piece of furniture, spread your legs apart, wider than hip width. Turn your feet out and bend your knees a few inches. Your stance should be comfortable and relaxed—in a plié position. Extend your left arm out away from you. This is Count 1.

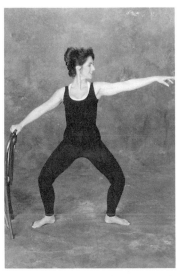

1.

2. Pull your left leg in to what's called a "coupé," or cupping, position. You'll be slightly crossing your left foot or to the far side of your right ankle, with your toes pressed lightly into the floor as you see here. Your right leg and right arm on the barre are supporting most of your weight. Now stretch your left arm up and over your head, reaching in a relaxed curve toward the barre. This is Count 2. Feel the stretch along the left side of your torso. Go back to the starting position of step 1. That will be count 3.

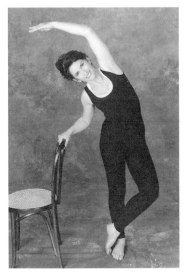

2.

(continued on next page)

3. Repeat the same coupé movement, but this time put your left foot behind your right leg. Stretch your left arm up and over your head. This is Count 4. Go back to the starting position. That will be Count 5.

4. This time, you'll bend your left knee and slide your foot up your shin—in what's called a "passé" movement. Extend your left arm out to the side, at shoulder height. This is Count 6. Keep your balance, and your body relaxed. Go back to the starting position. That will be Count 7.

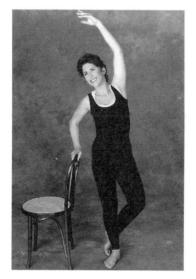

3.

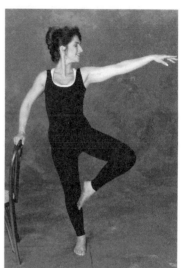

4.

5. This time, extend your left leg out to the side, about a foot off the floor. Try to keep this leg as straight as possible, but do not arch your back. Only lift it as high as you can without losing your position. Extend your left arm out to the side, at shoulder height. Your torso is erect yet relaxed. This is Count 8.

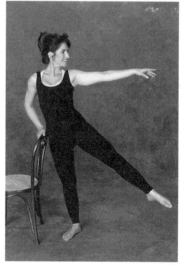

5.

14. Hamstring Stretch at the Barre — *Repetitions: Hold this stretch for at least 30–60 seconds on each side.*

1. Stand facing your barre or sturdy piece of furniture, then place the instep of your right foot up on it. Keep your left leg relaxed and knee bent very slightly. Lean into the barre, placing your arms comfortably on your right thigh. You'll feel the stretch in your left hip flexor and your right hamstring. These are Counts 1–4.

2. Gently bring your torso up and away from the barre. Try to straighten your right leg, but do not force this stretch. As you straighten your back, your arms will lift up simultaneously, palms facing each other. Inhale deeply. These are Counts 5–8. Keep your movements slow and controlled.

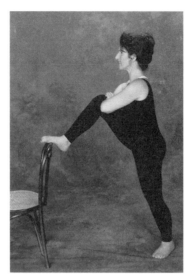 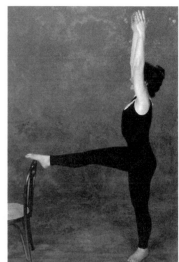

1. 2.

Callanetics Portion   (half an hour)

(see The Callanetics Basic Routine in chapter 5 for instructions)

Number of Repetitions

Legs

1. Pelvic Wave Leg Strengthener   *2 sets*
2. Standing Pelvic Rotations   *5 on each side*
3. Standing Front Thigh Stretch   *25 counts on each leg*

Arms, Waist, and Neck

4. Underarm Tightener—Sitting   *75*
5. Waist Away—Sitting   *75*
6. Neck Relaxer—Sitting   *1 set of 5 repetitions*

Hips and Behind

7. Bringing Up the Rear—Sitting   *75 on each side*
8. Out to the Side—Sitting   *75 on each side*

Inner Thigh Squeeze

9. Arches   *Count of 75*
10. Heels   *Count of 75*

Stomach

11. Open and Close   *20*
12. Single Leg Raise   *75 with each leg*
13. Double Leg Raise   *75*

Stretches

14. Inner Thigh Stretch   *30 seconds–1 minute*
15. Hamstring Stretch—Lying down   *30 seconds–1 minute for each leg*
16. Spine Stretch   *30 seconds–1 minute on each side*

SPECIAL ROUTINES AND MAINTENANCE PLANS

No matter what your physical condition, if your doctor has given you the go-ahead to exercise, chances are that gentle and safe Callanetics can help you. In this section I'm listing the relevant modifications, for each specific condition, to the Basic Routine of Chapter 5. I've only listed the exercises where there is some change; if the exercise itself is not listed, it means there is no change.

Arthritis

Fatigue and arthritis often go together, unfortunately, which is why an exercise routine that will improve your energy and sense of well-being is so crucial. Although you should never exercise during an acute flare-up, Callanetics is a perfect way to regain flexibility and improve your muscle tone without stressing those painful joints. Just start a regime very gradually, no more than ten to fifteen minutes total at first. If you're not in too much pain, try to do at least a few of the Callanetics exercises each day, as they can certainly increase your range of motion. Triple slow motion is more important than ever; jerky or quick movements can really cause pain.

Follow these tips if you have arthritis:

1. A long warm-up is critical. Move slowly, at your own pace.

2. Take a breather—*often.*

3. Really focus on your arthritic joints during the stretches. Relax into the position. Let your muscles stretch—don't you stretch your muscles! You never have to tense to get into a stretch.

4. Since you might have limited flexibility, you can do some of the standing exercises while seated. See page 189, "Never Exercised Before," for other specific tips.

5. Take a day or two off between sessions if you're in any pain. Don't ever push yourself if something hurts during a session. Stop—take a breather—relax. Having arthritis means you're used to chronic pain, but you should never try to work through the pain. Don't compare yourself with anyone else who may find simple movements much easier to do than you.

6. If your medication changes, be sure to discuss with your doctor any changes you may need to make in your exercise routine.

7. A long cooldown is just as critical as a long warm-up. Move slowly, at your own pace.

Bad Back and Posture Improvement

As you know, I wrote *Callanetics for Your Back* for the millions of us who suffer from back pain. Callanetics exercises not only stretch your back but effectively work your abdominal muscles. Often, lower-back pain comes from weak muscles; strengthen them and you'll automatically help improve your back. As ever, be sure to speak to your doctor or chiropractor before starting any routine. Remember:

1. Always warm up before exercising.

2. Get up from the floor gracefully (see p. 131). Always bend your knees when you're picking anything up or bending down. Think before you move!

3. Never skip abdominals because you feel they're hard to do. You need these more than ever.

4. Always cool down after exercising. Stretch those muscles.

Here is some of the routine, with modifications, done in Callanetics studios' Back Class. The repetition count is the same:

Warm-ups:

Up and Down

Swing

Underarm Tightener

Waist Away   Round shoulders forward.

Neck Relaxers   Curl your pelvis.

Stomach Exercises:

Bent-Knee Reach

Leg Exercises:

Pelvic Wave Leg   Go up and down twice.

Strengtheners   Keep your shoulders rounded.

Hamstring Stretch—Up and Over

Buttocks—Hips—Outer Thighs:

Bringing Up the Rear—Sitting,

Leg Bent

Out to the Side—Sitting

These can also be done standing, with pelvis curled up

Stretches:

Inner Thigh Stretch—Sitting   Do not take your legs far out to

Hamstring Stretch—Lying-down   the side.

Spine Stretch

Pelvis—Front and Inner Thighs:

Pelvic Rotations

Front Thigh Stretch

In addition, you can add these stretches at the end:

Stretch the entire back **Back Stretches**

1. Lie on the floor, with your knees bent, feet on the floor hip width apart, arms relaxed at your sides. Stretch the muscles at the back of your neck as if you were going to flatten it on the floor, then relax. Keep your jaw relaxed.

2. Press the small of your back into the floor by tightening your buttocks muscles.

3. Gently curl your pelvis up toward your navel. Hold for a count of 5, then release in triple slow motion to the floor. Each time curl up even more than you think you can, hold again for a count of 5, and release. Keep your entire body relaxed.

Repetitions: Work up to 5 sets

1. In the same position, slowly raise your right knee up to your chest. Place your hands in front of your leg below your knee or in back of your thigh. Gently hug your knee to your chest. Hold for a count of 5.

2. Lower your leg in triple slow motion. Repeat with the left leg.

Repetitions: Work up to 5 sets

1. In the same position, raise both knees, one at a time, to your chest. Place your hands in front of your legs below your knees, or hold the backs of your thighs, and gently hug your knees to your chest. Hold for a count of 5. Pull just enough to feel that your lower back is stretching and your tailbone is coming up slightly off the floor.

2. Slowly bring your legs down toward the floor, one at a time, keeping your knees bent.

Repetitions: Work up to 5 sets

Spinal Twist

Stretches spine, chest, shoulders, neck, between the shoulder blades; expands lungs

1. Sit on the floor, with your right leg stretched out straight in front of you. Place your left hand on the floor behind you, and rest your weight on it. Bend your left leg and cross over your right leg, knee facing the ceiling, resting your foot on the floor to the outside of your right knee. Stretch your torso up even higher.

2. Bend your right elbow and press your upper arm against the outside of your left knee. Slowly turn your head toward the left and gently try to look over your left shoulder, while turning your upper torso toward your left hand.

3. Reverse and repeat on the other side.

Repetitions: Hold for a count of 60 on each side

Do not hold your breath.

Do not arch your back.

Relax your entire body. Feel the lovely stretch.

Bridging

Stretches spine and neck; contracts buttocks and thigh muscles; contracts abdominals

1. Lie on your back with your knees bent, legs hip width apart, feet flat on the floor. Your arms are at your sides, palms down on the floor. Stretch your neck and pull in your chin.

2. Tighten your buttocks and curl up your pelvis. Keep curling your pelvis more than you think you can until your hips and buttocks lift up off the floor. (It's okay if your knees fall off a little to the sides.) With your pelvis still curled, raise your buttocks until your entire back is stretched straight. Your weight will be evenly distributed between your feet and your shoulders.

3. Slowly return your torso to the floor, one vertebra at a time. When you are flat on the floor, uncurl your pelvis.

Repetitions: Hold for a count of 60

Do not rest your weight solely on your shoulders.

Do not arch your back or crunch your neck.

Your feet are as light as feathers on the floor.

Do not tense your shoulders. Your entire body is relaxed.

Bad Knees

If you're familiar with the Basic Routine, you'll see that I've often indicated where you should place a mat or towel under your knees to prevent strain. Be sure to do the same here.

Warm-ups:

Up and Down	Barely bend your knees.
Swing	Barely bend your knees.

Leg Exercises:

Pelvic Wave Leg Strengtheners	Don't lower your body very far; take your body back; stand on your whole foot, with your feet apart.
Pliés	Don't lower your body very far; move your body back; stand on your whole foot, with your feet apart.

Buttocks—Hips—Outer Thighs:

Bringing Up the Rear—Sitting, Leg Bent	Straighten your leg a bit, and keep your knees relaxed.
Out to the Side—Sitting	Bend your leg a bit, and keep your leg relaxed.

Stretches:

Inner Thigh Stretch—Sitting	Bend your knees a little.

Pelvis—Front and Inner Thighs:

Pelvic Rotations	Place padding under your knees; move your upper body forward; if you feel it in your knees, try this standing at the barre.

Pelvic Scoop	Place padding under your knees; do not curl so much, or take your body all the way down; if you feel it in your knees, try this standing at the barre.
Front Thigh Stretch	Move your knees apart; do this standing up if you need to (see p. 154).
Inner Thigh Squeeze	Bend your knees slightly.

Bad Neck

If your neck is sore or easily strained, it's very important to do all your Callanetics exercises in a very relaxed manner. Always cradle the back of your head with both hands when doing any of the Stomach exercises.

Warm-ups:

Underarm Tightener	Concentrate on relaxing your neck.
Neck Relaxers	Do in triple slow motion.

Stomach Exercises:

Bent-Knee Reach	Do all the stomach exercises as follows: Cradle your head, elbows out to the side; or place pillows under your neck and shoulders if you need more cushioning.
Single Leg Raise	
Double Leg Raise	

Pelvis—Front and Inner Thighs:

Pelvic Rotations	Place your hands on your hips if you tend to tense your neck and shoulders for the Pelvic Rotations and Scoop.
Pelvic Scoop	

Dizziness and Circulatory Problems

If you have circulatory problems or high blood pressure, calm, steady, and even breathing is a must. Never strain or hold your breath. Always work at your own pace—if you can only do a few reps, don't worry. Each time you do Callanetics you'll be getting stronger. If your doctor advises you to keep your head elevated, always place a pillow under your head when doing any of the lying-down exercises.

Warm-ups:

Up and Down	Don't bend so far forward and keep your head up.
Swing	Don't bend so far forward and keep your head up.

Leg Exercises:

Hamstring Stretch—Up and Over	Do not do this exercise.

Fitness Rut

If you've found yourself in a fitness rut, you can take a long breather away from Callanetics exercises, for a week or so. After that amount of time it's easier to look back at what was bothering you and put it in perspective. Still, it is hard to be in a Callanetics rut—compared to other exercise routines—because you see such fast results. I've found that people who are frustrated often are not relaxing. Callanetics classes teach students to learn to relax, and then all of a sudden they realize the exercises feel flowing and completely different. Beginning students, for example, are tense—then all of a sudden they feel how deeply Callanetics works their muscles while they're in a relaxed state. Being tense is a waste of your energy.

Concentrate on your breathing and learning to relax. Take frequent breathers if you need to. Let yourself melt into the floor.

Hip Replacement

You might not believe this, but one of our best teachers has had a hip replacement. This woman is a perfect example of how a positive attitude and determination to "feel young" has not only aided her recuperation but also improved the quality of her life after major surgery. Just take a look at the high kicks of Liza Minelli and you'd never think she's had hip replacement surgery.

You don't need to make too many changes in the routine once your doctor gives you the go-ahead to resume exercising. If you feel any twinges, take a breather. Always check that your positions are correct.

Buttocks—Hips—Outer Thighs:

Bringing Up the Rear— Sitting, Leg Bent Out to the Side—Sitting	If you have any pain or pressure in your hip joint, lean all the way over to the side.

Never Exercised Before

If you've never exercised before or are elderly or out of shape, then you'll be doing the beginner's routine as shown in chapter 5. Here are additional tips:

Warm-ups:

Up and Down	Use very small movements.
Swing	Use very small movements.
Standing Hamstring Stretch	Lean on something if you need to; do not stay down so long.
Neck Relaxers	Do these sitting in a chair if you become dizzy.

Stomach Exercises:

Bent-Knee Reach

For all these, do low repetitions. Place a pillow under your head and shoulders.

Single Leg Raise

Cradle your head with your elbows out to the side.

Double Leg Raise

Hold on to your legs—you don't have to release; keep your arms parallel to the floor.

Leg Exercises:

Pelvic Wave Leg Strengtheners

Stand on your whole foot and don't bend your knees very far.

Pliés

Stand on your whole foot and don't bend your knees very far.

Hamstring Stretch—Up and Over

Place your heel on a lower barre or chair. Hold on to something for balance.

Buttocks—Hips—Outer Thighs:

Bringing Up the Rear—Sitting, Leg Bent

Lean over to the left side as far as necessary.

Out to the Side—Sitting

Lean over to the left side as far as necessary.

The Entire Body:

Open and Close

Drag your feet along the floor; bring your knees up into your chest; scoot farther away from the wall.

Stretches:

Sitting Inner Thigh Stretch

Do not move your legs so far to the side.

Sitting Hamstring Stretch	Do not round so far forward; bend your knees both up toward the ceiling, or keep one leg bent in front; do this standing or lying down if more comfortable.

Pelvis—Front and Inner Thighs:

Pelvic Rotations	Hold on to the barre for more support; move your upper body forward for better balance; do this standing up if that's easier.
Pelvic Scoop	Hold on to the barre for more support; do this standing up if that's easier.
Front Thigh Stretch	Lean back for better balance; do this standing up.

Posture

Once Callanetics has taught you proper alignment, your posture will automatically improve. And you'll never have to worry about stooping forward or developing a "dowager's hump." The most important exercises to improve your posture are in the Warm-up section. Try to do the Underarm Tightener, Waist Away, and Neck Relaxers every day.

Pregnancy and Postpartum

When you're pregnant, you gain weight and retain fluid; your center of gravity shifts; your hormone levels change; and your joints loosen and lubricate in preparation for delivery, so extra care when doing any exercises is a must. That doesn't mean you should stop exercising altogether, of course! If you're having any complications with your pregnancy, or just experiencing low energy and feeling blah, be sure to consult your obstetrician or health-care professional for the best advice about your exercise routines.

As the warning in the front of this book states, you must never do any of the stomach exercises in your first trimester. Your doctor can best advise you.

I recommend that you wait at least six weeks after delivery to resume a Callanetics routine. Follow these modifications pre- and post-baby.

Warm-ups:

Hamstring Stretch	Lean on something when you do this stretch; do not stay down as long.

Stomach Exercises:

As you know, Callanetics stomach exercises should never be done in the first trimester. Starting around the end of your second trimester, do all your stomach exercises from a sitting position—but *only* if you are very experienced with the entire SuperCallanetics program. Take frequent breathers.

Leg Exercises:

Pelvic Wave Leg Strengtheners	Stand on your whole foot; don't bend your knees very far.
Pliés	Stand on your whole foot; don't bend your knees very far
Hamstring Stretch—Up and Over	Place your heel on a lower barre; hold on to something for balance.

Buttocks—Hips—Outer Thighs:

Bringing Up the Rear—Sitting, Knee Bent	Lean over to the left side as far as necessary.
Out to the Side—Sitting	Lean over to the left side as far as necessary.

The Entire Body:

Open and Close	*Do not do this exercise!*

Stretches:

Lying Down Hamstring Stretch	After about 5 months, do instead: Hamstring Stretch—Up and Over (as modified above).
Spine Stretch	Do the Spinal Twist instead (in Bad Back section, above).

Pelvis—Front and Inner Thighs:

Pelvic Rotations	Do them standing at the barre.
Pelvic Scoop	Do this standing at the barre.
Front Thigh Stretch	Do this standing at the barre.

Recuperation from Surgery

Once your doctor has given you the go-ahead to begin an exercise regime, you should always proceed with caution and common sense. (With all my back problems before Callanetics, believe me—I know!) Although it may be tempting, don't try to do too much at once, or you could injure yourself. Take it slow, keep it gentle, in triple slow motion, and if you feel fatigued, then take a breather, or try again the next day.

It's especially important to begin exercises as soon as you can to improve your energy and circulation. Even if you're an experienced Callanetics student, always go back to a beginner's routine until you feel strong enough to move on to your regular routine. Always listen to your body!

Callanetics 15-Minute Maintenance Plan

If your schedule is particularly hectic, or you're traveling, here's a quick program that I designed to work on the areas that need the most help. Don't leave anything out! Add a few of your favorite exercises if you have more time. And don't forget—even if you're stuck in an airport waiting for your flight to leave, you can brace yourself against a chair and perform a leg exercise or two. (Not only will this get your circulation going, but it'll also help you stay comfortable if you're seated next to the kind of zany travelers I always seem to get stuck next to!)

Warm-ups:

Up and Down	Repeat 5 times.
Underarm Tightener	Do 75.
Waist Away	Do 75 on each side.

Stomach Exercises:

Bent-Knee Reach	Do 75.
Single Leg Raise	Do 75.

Leg Exercises:

Pelvic Wave Leg Strengthener	Do 5 sets.
Hamstring Stretch #1 — Up and Over	Do each side for 30 seconds.

Buttocks—Hips—Outer Thighs:

Bringing Up the Rear—Sitting, Leg Bent	Do 75 on each side.
Bringing Up the Rear—Sitting, Leg Straight	Do 75 on each side.

Stretches:

Sitting Hamstring Stretch	Do this for 30 seconds.

Pelvis—Front and Inner Thighs:

Pelvic Scoop	Do 8.
Inner Thigh Squeeze.	Hold for a count of 100.

RESOURCES

American Association of
Retired People
601 W Street, NW
Washington, DC 20049
(202) 434-2277

American Cancer Society
1-800-422-6237

American Dental Association
211 E. Chicago Ave.
Chicago, IL 60611
(312) 440-2500

American Lung Association
1-800-USA-LUNG

Center for Anxiety and
Stress Treatment
4350 Executive Dr., Suite 204
San Diego, CA 92121
(619) 458-1066/Fax: (619) 542-0730

Center for Medical Consumers
237 Thompson St.
New York, NY 10012
(212) 674-7105

Consumer Information Center
(U.S. Government)
P.O. Box 100
Pueblo, CO 81002
(719) 948-3334

National Alliance of Breast Cancer
Organizations
1180 Sixth Ave.
New York, NY 10036
(212) 719-0154

National Cancer Institute
1-800-4CANCER

The National Center for
Homeopathy
801 N. Fairfax #306
Alexandria, VA 22314
(703) 548-7790

National Heart, Lung, and
Blood Institute
9000 Rockville Pike
Building 31, Room 4A-21
Bethesda, MD 20892
(301) 951-3260

National Institute on Aging
1-800-222-2225

National Women's Health Network
1325 G Street, NW, Lower Level
Washington, DC 20077-2052
(202) 293-6045

National Women's Health
Resource Center
2440 M Street, NW, Suite 325
Washington, DC 20037
(202) 293-6045

North American Menopause Society
University Hospitals of Cleveland
2074 Abington Rd.
Cleveland, OH 44106
(216) 844-3334

The North American Vodder
Association of Lymphatic
Therapy (Ayurvedic)
c/o Howard Douglass
P.O. Box 861
Chesterland, OH 44026

Older Women's League
666 11th Street, NW Suite 700
Washington, DC 20001
(202) 783-6686

SMOKENDERS
1-800-243-5614

Women's Action Alliance
370 Lexington Ave., Suite 603
New York, NY 10017
(212) 532-8330

SUGGESTED READING

Ackerman, Diane. *A Natural History of the Senses*. New York: Random House, 1990.

Andes, Karen. *A Woman's Book of Strength: An Empowering Guide to Total Mind/Body Fitness*. New York: Perigee, 1995.

Bailey, Covert. *The New Fit or Fat*. Boston: Houghton Mifflin, 1977, 1978, 1991.

Cooper, Kenneth. *Preventing Osteoporosis*. New York: Bantam, 1989.

Cutler, W., and Garcia, C. *Menopause: A Guide for Women and the Men Who Love Them*. New York: Norton, 1992.

Darden, Ellington. *Living Longer Stronger*. New York: Perigee, 1995.

Doress, Paula Brown, and Siegal, Diana Laskin. *Ourselves, Growing Older: Women Aging with Knowledge and Power*. New York: Touchstone, 1987.

Evans, William, Rosenberg, Irwin H., and Thompson, Jacqueline. *Biomarkers, The 10 Determinants of Aging You Can Control*. New York: Simon & Schuster, 1991.

Greer, Germaine. *The Change: Women, Aging, and the Menopause*. New York: Fawcett Columbine, 1991.

Healthy People 2000: National Health Promotion and Disease Prevention Objectives; U.S. Department of Health and Human Services/Public Health Service, U.S. Government Printing Office, 1990.

Helfant, Dr. Richard H. *The Woman's Guide to Fighting Heart Disease*. New York: Perigee, 1993.

Landau, Carol, Cyr, Michele, and Moulton, Anne. *The Complete Book of Menopause*. New York: Perigee, 1994.

Laurence, Leslie, and Weinhouse, Beth. *Outrageous Practices: The Alarming Truth about How Medicine Mistreats Women*. New York: Fawcett Columbine, 1994.

Moyers, Bill. *Healing and the Mind.* New York: Bantam Doubleday Dell, 1993.

Padus, Emrika. *The Complete Guide to Your Emotions and Your Health.* Emmaus, Pa.: Rodale, 1992.

Pashkow, Dr. Fredric J., and Libov, Charlotte. *The Woman's Heart Book: The Complete Guide to Keeping Your Heart Healthy and What to Do If Things Go Wrong.* New York: Penguin, 1993.

Rechelbacher, Horst. *Rejuvenation: A Wellness Guide for Women and Men.* Rochester, Vt.: Healing Arts Press, 1987, 1989.

Rose, Jeanne. *The Aromatherapy Book.* Berkeley, Calif.: North Atlantic, 1992.

——. *Jeanne Rose's Modern Herbal.* New York: GD/Perigee, 1987.

Sheehy, Gail. *The Silent Passage.* New York: Random House, 1991.

Waterhouse, Debra. *Outsmarting the Female Fat Cell.* New York: Hyperion, 1993.

White, Augustus A., III. *Your Aching Back: A Doctor's Guide to Relief.* New York: Fireside, 1983, 1990.

CALLANETICS STUDIOS NEAR YOU

There are over sixty certified Callanetics exercise studios internationally. Only teachers trained by a Master Teacher who works directly with me are certified to teach Callanetics exercises. For further information on studios located in your area, call 1-800-8-CALLAN.

INDEX